KNOW THYSELF

Attain to Happiness & Live a Good Life

Dr. A.P. Sharma

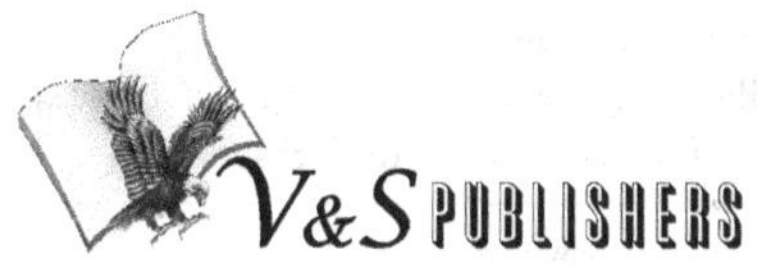

Published by:

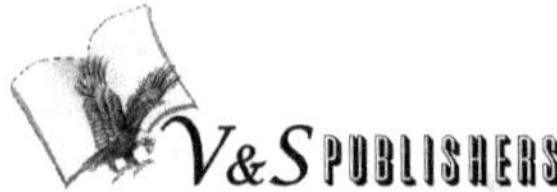

F-2/16, Ansari road, Daryaganj, New Delhi-110002
☎ 23240026, 23240027 • *Fax:* 011-23240028
Email: info@vspublishers.com • *Website:* www.vspublishers.com

Branch : Hyderabad
5-1-707/1, Brij Bhawan (Beside Central Bank of India Lane)
Bank Street, Koti Hyderabad - 500 095
☎ 040-24737290
E-mail: vspublishershyd@gmail.com

Distributors :

- **Pustak Mahal**®, Delhi
  J-3/16, Daryaganj, New Delhi-110002
  ☎ 23276539, 23272783, 23272784 • *Fax:* 011-23260518
  E-mail: sales@pustakmahal.com • *Website:* www.pustakmahal.com
  Bengaluru: ☎ 080-22234025 • *Telefax:* 22240209
  Patna: ☎ 0612-3294193 • *Telefax:* 0612-2302719
- **PM Publications**
  - 10-B, Netaji Subhash Marg, Daryaganj, New Delhi-110002
    ☎ 23268292, 23268293, 23279900 • *Fax:* 011-23280567
    *E-mail:*rapidexdelhi@indiatimes.com, pmpublications@gmail.com
  - 6686, Khari Baoli, Delhi-110006
    ☎ 23944314, 23911979
- **Unicorn Books**
  Mumbai :
  23-25, Zaoba Wadi (Opp. VIP Showroom), Thakurdwar, Mumbai-400002
  ☎ 22010941 • *Telefax:* 022-22053387

ISBN 978-93-813845-1-0

Edition : 2011

Price : ₹ 120/-

Printed at : Param Offsetters, Okhla, New Delhi-110020

Dedicated to

Shri Jiddu Krishnamurti

Preface

Began to contemplate on the theme around two and a half years back when my book titled, *J.Krishnamurti: His Concept of Freedom* was published. After giving much thought to it and going through the related literature for a considerable time, I started working on it in the early 1996. Several obstacles came on my way as I learnt about the Self, the more obscure it appeared to me. Perhaps, the only way to know it could be to talk to people about it, and to read more. I, therefore, talked to people. I interviewed, through an unstructured procedure, around 350 educated people in India, England and in the United States and tried to gather their opinion about what they thought of the Self. The interviews did not reveal more as most people said that they would think about it and reply later. Obviously, they did not. If some did say anything, their answers were fragmentary or religiously and culturally biased. I could not get a clear meaning of the Self. Then I tried to dig more into the philosophical books—both Western and Eastern. I found that philosophers such as Plato, Aristotle and others in the West, and Buddha, Samkara and Krishnamurti in the East, did define the Self to a great extent.

It was simply an immense pleasure to know about it—especially through the examples quoted by Plato and the Buddhist masters' and monks' discourses. The first chapter of the book, therefore, talks about 'The meaning of the Self', including my own reflections on 'Why do we need to know the Self?'

The purpose of the book was not merely to know the characteristics of the Self. It was also to find out the meaning 'To Know Thyself' as well as to learn the process 'How to Attain that Knowledge.' Only then the individual would be able to get more in touch with himself and would discover his selfishness, vagueness, hatred, anger, fear and diversity, that he cradles everyday in his life. If the Self is pure and if it possesses spiritual and virtuous qualities as Plato and other ancient philosophers contended, why it would ever possess unvirtuous thoughts? The truth is that the Self often experiences those odd feelings too and plunges into gloom and disharmony. Does it mean that the duality is real and one's getting deluded is natural?

The deluded Self is bound to leap into some kind of disharmony, resulting in breeding hatred, fear, selfishness and anger. Therefore, after knowing the meaning of the Self, it seemed to me imperative that one must also know 'Why does the Self often feel divided and deluded?' It led me to believe that the duality about which Plato, Aristotle, Samkara and the Gita talked, was not totally unreal?

I then contended that if one knew the nature of duality and understood the process that crystallized it, it would be easier to decipher the cause of the unvirtuous thoughts. Therefore, to learn the views of the philosophers it was very important as they could help clarifying the meaning of dualism. The second chapter contains all that.

The third and the fourth chapters provide explanations that duality (diversity) can be dissolved by attaining the unity of the Self. The divided Self, implicit with mean desires such as envy, fear, hatred, dissolution, lust and anger, may get rid of them and be united with its pure Self. To reach that goal one requires to follow a simple process that involves self-reflection and a balanced state of mind. In light of that, some important ideas have been presented to help the mind, decipher its meaning and base inclinations. Those ideas are highly inspirational and can help transcending to a higher plane without accomplishing big practices.

The book has some more important landmarks. These are:

1. Buddhist masters' and monks' lively discussions have been quoted to highlight the meaning of the Self. The style of the discourses is so natural and fascinating that the reader cannot escape enjoying them.
2. Comparative views of the Eastern and Western philosophers have been presented to clarify the meaning of the Self. Adequate quotes have been provided to make reading more attractive.
3. Some good examples, similes and myths have been quoted from the writings of the great masters to make their viewpoints more interesting and clear.

4. As some formal research was also made to discover the meaning of the Self, the material will surely be of great help to students of philosophy and education at the under-graduate level in most universities and countries.

The issue to understand the knowledge of the Self is very obscure. Yet the ideas presented in the book are not only lucid but also highly inspirational. I hope that the reader, who is desirous to know about his turmoil and disharmony and wants to attain peace of mind, happiness and stability in life, will surely welcome my efforts.

16th January, 1999 **–A.P. Sharma**

Acknowledgement

For kind permission to reprint certain copyright material grateful acknowledgment is hereby made as follows: Krishnamurti Foundation of America Ojai, California; Krishnamurti Foundation Trust Limited Brockwood Park, Hamphshire, U.K.; Houghton Mifflin Company, Boston, Massachusetts; David Higam Associates Limited, London; Harper Collins Publishers, Hammersmith, London; Cliffs Notes Inc. Lincoln, NE, USA; Dover Publications, Inc. Mineola, NY; Central Chinmaya Mission Trust, Mumbi; Osho, International Foundation, NY.

Though every reasonable care has been taken to trace ownership of copyright material, information will be welcomed that will enable the publisher to rectify in the subsequent editions any incorrect or missing reference or credit.

Contents

1

What is the Self?

At times it seems difficult to get a clear meaning of a concept even though we feel that we know everything about it. In Shakespeare's Hamlet, when Ophelia's father asked Hamlet, "What is the meaning of madness?", Hamlet, after a brief pause, replied casually, "Madness is madness". Well, we can accept it simply as kidding on the part of Hamlet. But if we ask someone 'What is the meaning of the Self?', he may not be able to respond so quickly and casually. It would surely regulate a lot of thinking to give an acceptable answer. It really happened so. When I asked a good number of people, 'What they thought about the Self?', most of them ignored the question. If anyone answered the question it contained his religious or cultural bias. I expected an answer on metaphysical grounds. Most of them found it difficult to define it. Perhaps that is the reason that philosophers from ancient times seem to be religiously busy in evolving a convincing and acceptable definition of the Self.

Both, in the Western as well as Eastern worlds, the quest to know the Self has been very intensive. As they go on defining it, it often seems that a majority of them do not possess a very clear picture of it in their minds. Not really that they have not tried hard, but because it is so difficult to go deeper into the Self and know it. Therefore, on my journey to find out 'The Meaning to Know Thyself', my first milestone is to find out a clearer concept of the Self.

The Western Point of View

Greek Concern

In my quest to know the Self, I start by looking back at the scene, which took place in Athens some 400-500 years back, before the Christ. Socrates, accompanied by his friend Crito, is attempting to know from Mouse, the city potter, the meaning of beautiful.

Socrates asked, "What is this thing called beautiful, Mouse?"

"Beautiful," said Mouse, and looked puzzled for a minute, and touched the shoulder of the pot he had been making. "Why like this, I suppose, and like that one over there..." Socrates put his hand on the pot, too, to feel the curve of it, but it seemed clear that he was not satisfied. "No, Mouse, not that way! That's what people always do—points at things. They point at things and say, 'Beautiful this, beautiful that', and the things are all different. Beautiful pot, beautiful wrestling, beautiful courage—all different. But what is the sameness of them? There must be a sameness somehow."

Mouse did not answer right away. At last, after some time, he said, "I don't know about 'the beautiful', Socrates. I only know about good pots. A good pot is a beautiful pot to me."

"But why is it good, Mouse?" Socrates asked him.

"See that pitcher over there?" Mouse said, pointing again "That is a good pitcher. It is good for something. It is good for pouring. Make the lip a little more deeply curved and wine will spill. Make the sides a little fatter and it will tip over easily. Then it is a bad pitcher. In fact, to my way of thinking, unless it does the thing that it is supposed to do it can hardly be called a pitcher at all..."

"Then it must be the goodness in things that makes them beautiful and useful. It must be the goodness in them that makes them anything at all," Socrates said slowly.[1] Perhaps that was the beginning of the dawn of knowledge in him. He went on and on with his search for truth until he discovered that just being alive was not the important thing, but living rightly. For that he never compromised with truth, even at the cost of his life. It is because of that, the philosophic Europe has always considered Socrates such a great teacher.

Some eminent thinkers believe that had Socrates been born in

India, he would certainly have been looked upon as an 'Avatar', an incarnation of Godhead. If he had been born in Palestine or Arabia, he would have figured as a Prophet of God, for he had something special in him that distinguished him from all ordinary persons. He claimed to be guided by an Oracle or sign, a kind of voice, which always forbade but did not command.[2]

He was known to be subject to trances. *Symposium* records that one morning he could not find a solution of what he was thinking. So he stood still in thoughts from early dawn till noon. As crowd gathered round him, he continued standing, lost in thoughts until the next morning.[3]

Socrates' glory lies in his pertinacity with which he fought the battle of liberty of thought and the supremacy of righteousness in life, with such courage that he defied death. His message has come down to us through centuries. Who could utter such words other than him as he possessed the soul of a true and good person. He reflects:

> *I believe that no great good has ever happened in the State than my service to the God. For I do nothing but persuading you all, old and young alike, not to take thought for your persons, or your properties, but first and chiefly care about the greatest improvement of the soul. I tell you that virtue is not given by money but that from virtue comes money and every other good of man, public I believe that no greater good has ever happened in the state than my service as well as private.*[4]

The *Apology* unfolds that Socrates brought to his fellow citizens some special message from God. It was that it is the great business of life to practise the 'care' or 'tendencies' of one's soul, to make it as good as possible. No one should ruin one's life as most people do by caring for the body or for 'possessions' before caring for the soul. Socrates reflects that the fundamental thought is that the *soul is most truly a man's self*. Socrates defined it as the normal waking personality, the seat of character and intelligence, "that in virtue of which we are called wise or foolish, good or bad".

Consequently, the thought works out that "the soul is the man".* Our happiness or well being, therefore, depends directly on the goodness or badness of the soul. Socrates contends that there is no happiness in possessing health, or strength or wealth, unless one knows how to use these advantages rightly. He continues, 'if we use them wrongly they will lead us to different kinds of misery.' This leads us to understand that the good state of the soul is precisely that state in which it never makes the mistake of taking anything to be good when it is not really good. To make one's soul as good as possible one needs to attain the knowledge of good that will prevent him from using strength, health, wealth and opportunity wrongly.**

According to a famous myth which Socrates relates to Phaedrus on the bank of the Ilissus, the soul, in its original state, can be compared to a chariot drawn by two-winged horses. One is docile but thoroughbred. The other is a governable steed (the passion and sensuous instincts). This chariot is driven by a charioteer (reason) who strives to guide it properly. In a region above heaven the chariot travels through the world of the Ideas, which the soul thus contemplates, although not without difficulty. Trouble arises in guiding the flight of the two horses, and the soul falls, the horses lose their wings and the soul becomes incarnated in the body. [5]

Most primitive people thought of the soul as a kind of shadowy image or replica of the body—like vapour or breath. They thought it was capable of leaving the body during sleep and surviving it after death. Greek literature and philosophy are permeated with the idea of the soul as expressed by the Greek word, 'psyche'. It carries a rich connotation of life, soul and consciousness. The earliest Greek thinkers believed in a "divine and animate essence", immanent in nature, appearing in a person as the soul, the source of life and intelligence. This view found expression in Heraclitus's doctrines. He thought that soul is a fiery vapour, which is identical with rational and vital fire-soul of the universe.[6] The tendency towards the complete spiritualization of the soul leading to an uncompromising dualism, is observed in Plato and later on in the teaching of Saint Auguistine. Gradually it emerged into the doctrine of the existence of the two worlds, a mundane, material world, and a divine spiritual world. The body

* In the later Academic formulations a man a soul using a body.

** Quoted from Encyclopedia Britannica, Vol. 12, pp. 919–920.

belongs to the former and the soul to the later.

Truly speaking, after Socrates, Plato's description of the soul, is more distinctive. Socrates went on telling us more about the goodness and badness of the soul rather than about its nature. For Plato, the soul is an immaterial essence or being, imprisoned in the body, its nature having little in common with the earthly, its home and destiny being the world of eternal Ideas. They correspond with what we now refer to as reason, will and feeling. The latter two are close to the physical body and evidently are not immortal. The reason is the 'divine' part of the soul is separate and as independent from the body. Thus, Plato characterized the soul as having both, the mortal and immortal qualities. It has also been discovred by him in his 'Simile of the Cave ' in the *Republic*. Aristotle emphasizes the reality and essential character of the soul not less than Plato, but he brings it into much closer relation to the body. He considers it the very 'form' and reality and perfection of the body. It is, according to Aristotle, the 'primary actuality of a natural body' endowed with life. The *Nicomachean Ethics* is probably the most popular of all Aristotle's works, which consists of a search analysis of the human character and conduct and every reader may find in it some picture of himself. In it, he desired every one of us to search for the 'good' that he identifies with happiness. What then is happiness and how do we achieve it?

According to Aristotle, every creature is happy fulfilling just the functions for which nature designed him. In the case of an individual, his unique function is the activity of the soul in obedience to reason. Virtues for us then are states of character in which we choose our activities rationally and therefore properly. It is through virtues that we may arrive at the state of happiness which we all so greatly desire.[7]

In the *Nicomachean Ethics*, in the eighth chapter, Aristotle defines 'good' as having three classes: external goods—external as they are called, goods of the soul, and goods of the body. Of these three classes, goods of the soul are considered goods in the strictest and truest sense. Spiritual actions and activities are ascribed to the soul. This theory, though ancient, is accepted by the philosophers of the present time too. It is correct, in the sense, that we call certain actions and activities the end, because we put the end in some good of the soul and not in an external good. 'By the similar theory a happy person lives well and does well. Happiness is, in fact, a kind of living and doing well... Now, most persons may find a sense of discord in their pleasure, because their pleasures are not all naturally pleasant. But the lovers of nobleness take pleasure, in what is naturally pleasant, and virtuous acts are naturally pleasant. Such acts are pleasant both to these people and to themselves. Therefore, happiness is always rooted in the soul that is both noble and good.'[8]

Elucidating further the meaning of the soul, Aristotle deals with it in his other book called by its Latin name, *De Anima*. Though it is a book on physics, Aristotle made his first systematic elaboration in it of the problem of the psyche. The essence of the soul is that it is a principle of life. For Aristotle, the life of an entity consists of its nourishment, growth and self-consumption. Thus, the soul is the 'form' or realization of a living body. The soul "informs" or gives form to the matter of a living thing, giving it its corporal being and making it a living body. Therefore, it is not a question of he soul's being superimposed on the body or added to it. Rather, the body is a living body because it has a soul. Aristotle states in *De Anima II* on page 1, that the soul is the realization of a natural organic body. He explains his point with the help of an example. He says that if the eye were a living creature, its soul would be its sight. The eye is the matter of sight, and if sight is missing, there is no relevance of an eye. As the eye is the physical eye united with the power of sight, so the soul and the body make up living thing.[9] Aristotle distinguishes different classes of souls. He professes that each living thing has only one soul, but human being, concretely, has a rational soul. It is the 'form' of his body. It was because of that he always professed that the form must be kept upright and be in possession of good thinking. It would lead a person to do good, that ultimately is the source of happiness.

European Contention

There have been thinkers in the Western world who have taken the soul as a collection of ideas or impressions only. For example, David Hume bluntly remarked that we have no experience of any such thing as a soul at all. We do not have any evidence for its existence. He thought that experience gave us nothing but a lot of impressions or perceptions and ideas or memory images. We had no way of showing or reason for believing that the soul is anything more than a collection of these impressions and ideas. He stated:

There are some philosophers who imagine we are every moment intimately conscious of what we call our self; that we feel its existence and its continuance in existence; and are certain, beyond the evidence of a demonstration, both of its perfect identity and simplicity... He continued further; For my part, when I enter most intimately into what I call myself, I always stumble on some particular perception or other, or heat or cold, light or shade, love or hatred, pain or pleasure. I never can catch myself at any time without perception, and never can observe anything but the perception, when my perceptions are removed for any time, as by sound sleep, so long am I insensible of myself, and may truly be said not to exist.[10]

Hume strongly believed that if anyone attempted to think seriously and without prejudice, he would never have a different notion of himself than what he had reflected. If any one did possess something different than what Hume had reflected, to him he would simply say that he may be right. At the same time Hume himself was also right, and that they both were essentially different too. He would have perceived something simple and continued, which he called himself; though Hume was certain that there was no such principle implicit in himself.[11]

What is meant by *self*, according to Hume is, that the Self is simply the totality of experiences and nothing more. These experiences are mostly conditioned and organized by principles of association, such as contiguity and resemblance. Kant once reflected that Hume was correct in saying that the Self was simply the totality of experiences but he did not go far enough in his analysis of the situation. He thought that there lied in the very nature of the case that the Self could never become the object of experience. The Self, whatever else that might be, was in the indefeasible situation of being the subject of experience. Knowledge of the Self seemed to be difficult in Kant's opinion. Well, without going into the subtleties and difficulties of Kant's position it seems safe to say that Kant was in no doubt at all as to the fact of there being a self. He also stated that what that self was, was beyond the possibility of knowledge.

William McDougall revived the use of the word *Animism.** It is the term he gave to his philosophy of mind, that is just his soul theory. He states that the mind, or if we choose to use the other terms, *soul, ego, self*—is a unitary and distinct psychic being. It is not wise to get identified or confused with body with which it interacts. In the absolute or objective system the whole universe is rooted and grounded in mind or spirit. One may call it Absolute Ego, as did Fichte, or Absolute Idea with Hegel, or Absolute Will with Schopenhaur or Absolute Experience with Bradley, or Absolute Self with Royce. The soul of person is, therefore, intimate with, or participates in, or represents the very essence of reality. Mind is not that which accompanies matter or which is generated by an evolutionary process, but it is primordial and original; it is the very stuff of the Universe.[12]

The foregoing discussion leads us to understand that the philosophers have often used the word mind to replace self or vice versa. To some, these terms—mind, soul or spirit—are absolutely synonymous but to others the mind is defined as a flux of consciousness. How far the mind and consciousness are akin or synonym ours, need some attention. We will take it up a little later. Let us first discuss briefly the various theories of mind that may help us to know a little more about the Self, which is the sole objective of this chapter.

Five Theories of Mind

In the history of philosophy, mind has been defined in different ways. It can be summarized under five theories of the mind. First it is the subjective theory held by Descartes who held that mind or soul is a separate, independent entity. Second, the epiphenomen-elastic theory, which states that mind is a kind of inefficacious by-product of the body. According to this theory, the soul would perish with the disintegration of the body and all so called mental or conscious life is reducible to the physical. The third theory denies a subjective mind and holds that what we mean by "mind" is nothing but a succession of experiences or mental states. This is Hume's point of view. The fourth is the functional view, such as the Aristotelian theory as well as those in recent times which hold that the mind is

* The word *animism* has been commonly used in anthropology to signify the tendency among primitive people to endow everything with mind, even things we regard as inanimate, such as stone and stick, etc. Mc Dougall uses the term in a large sense, merely to indicate belief in mind (anima), as reality.

an adaptive instrument developed or emerged in the long course of evolution. The fifth is the extreme behaviouristic type of theory that holds that mind at best is simply the behaviour of certain organisms. This theory even denies the mind but presents an account of it. Patric reflects whether the above theories lead us to conceive or not any clear philosophy of the mind, but surely in some measures they converse towards certain definite results. One of these conclusions is the Freudian emphasis upon vital impulses, those deep biological interests that seem like psychical energies that often drive us on apparently with some unconscious purpose. Yet there is another view that is familiar with the new movements. It is that what we call mental activity objectively considered, that kind of behaviour that we call adaptive. Warren has concluded that the belief is that adaptive behaviour has a subjective side that we may call *consciousness* or *experience*. There is another belief emphasized by Plato. He believes that there is peculiar unitary personal character of the Self. Finally Aristotle's point of view that considers mind as the perfection and fruition of the body. Aristotle's theory of mind as a dynamic entity, is closely bound up with the organism. It is receiving more serious attention, as is evident in such a movement as the Gestalt theory.[13]

We have already considered the views of the most prominent Western philosophers in the light of mind-body relationship. Let us also briefly consider, at this juncture, the relationship between mind and consciousness and wind up our discussion on the issue of the meaning of the Self from the Western point of view.

Patric reflects that philosophically we shouldn't use the word consciousness synonymous with the mind. We might say that something called consciousness accompanies all mental states and processes, but even this is questionable. Freudians have developed a vital as well as a widely accepted theory of mind, in which unconscious mental elements play an important part. For example, we may witness fear or anger in the child; they are simply fear and anger—not consciousness. If one reflects that one is conscious of the child's anger, it may mean nothing more than that one perceives fear or anger or is aware of it. The child himself may be conscious of his own anger, but if he is, the two are certainly not the same. Truly speaking, he may not be conscious of it. It is quite likely that he is not; he is just angry. Therefore, mind and consciousness are not the same.[14]

Let us stretch a little more about consciousness to make it further clear. Patric presents a beautiful example. Suppose one is sitting in a room where a clock is ticking. He is engaged in an interesting task and is not conscious of the clock. Suddenly, he becomes conscious of the clock ticking. That means simply that he becomes aware of it as his attention was drawn towards it. Thus, we see that consciousness in its simplest form is just awareness; it gradually takes on the relation of interest and meaning. Consciousness, thus, appears to be a special kind of relation between the percipient subject and the thing perceived. It is not the same for the whole mind; neither it is the same as mind nor soul. It is not even any special kind of stuff. Yet it is a distinct feature of that total thing we call mind or soul. Thus mind and consciousness are two different entities, but the latter is a property of the former and not entirely the former, that is mind or soul. Neither consciousness can be taken as the essence of life. Bertrand Russell, analyzing the term mind writes, 'Whatever may be the correct definition of consciousness, consciousness is not the essence of life. Nor we can think any longer of it as being a kind of substance or primordial stuff, out of which the world is made. We cannot even think of it as an entity or quality of being in itself.'[15]

Let us discuss a little more on the meaning of consciousness. Distinguishing mind with consciousness, Warren quite lucidly explains both. He says; 'Adaptive behaviour when witnessed in others we call mind; when experienced in ourselves, it is called consciousness. Conscious phenomena are simply mental phenomena as they appear subjectively in our own experience. Warren reflected that there are two ways of observing mental phenomena—in others and in ourselves; in the later case the mental phenomena form a group of conscious phenomena. Consciousness is thus a kind of privacy—an intimate, inner, serious aspect of mental life, only half revealed to the observation of others.[16] S. Alexander also endorses the same opinion about consciousness. He reflects that 'Consciousness is merely an experience, experienced by the one who possesses it and who is thinking, feeling, wondering and longing'.[17]

Eastern Approach

Vedantic *Saksin**

The Eastern approach, to identify the meaning of the Self, basically starts with the Vedantic philosophy. In fact, in Advaita the explanation

* Saks*in* means 'Witness or a disinterested looker-on'. The conception is thus relative, and the *saksin* as such is not, therefore, Brahman.

of the nature of the conscious element is almost the same as in the Sankhya-Yoga. It is conceived as extraneous to the apparatus, which yet in some way helps in manifestation and ultimately goes back eventually to the same source, viz., Brahman or Spirit. Like Sankhya-Yoga, in Advaita too the physical and the psychical are two distinct elements. The psychical element is viewed as wholly inactive. The activity it manifests only seemingly, belongs to it. In reality it needs to be traced to its physical accomplishment, viz., the internal organ. The element of conscious is known as *saksin*, which corresponds to *Purusha* of Sankhya-Yoga—the passive observer of the states of the internal organs as they unfold themselves. It appears never by itself, but always in association with the internal organ in its latent or manifest form. It is also true that no internal organ is conceivable without involving a reference to some *saksin* or other. Thus, it is only the unity of the passive *saksin* and the active *antah-karan* (internal organ) that is real for all purposes. That is what knows, feels and wills. In this complex form it is known as *jiva* or the empirical self. The double character of subject and object that are one and the same *jiva*, exhibits in so called self-consciousness.

This complex entity is believe to endure in one form or the other till the time of release. When at last it breaks up, the internal organs are absorbed by its sources, *Maya*. It is the same as the *prakrit* of the Sankhya-Yoga, as is also illustrated in the *Bhagvad Gita*. When the *saksin* loses its *saksi-hood*, it becomes Brahman indeed. The *saksin* and the *jiva* are not identical, though at the same time they are not quite different either. The *jiva* may become the object of self-consciousness on account of the objective element it includes. Yet it is wrong to speak of the *saksin* as knowable, for it is the pure element of awareness in all knowing. To assume that it is knowable, would be to imply another knowing element—a process that leads to the fallacy of infinite regress. But the sa*ksin* does not, therefore, remain unrealized, for being self-luminous, by its very nature, it does not require to be made known at all. In other words *jiva* is spirit as immanent in the *antah-karana*, while the *saksin* is spirit as transcendent.[18]

Gita's Conceptions

Before indulging in our search to know the meaning of the Self (soul) from the point of view of the modern Indian philosophers and certain schools of the Eastern philosophy,

I would like to explain its meaning as explained in the *Bhagwad Gita*. When Arjuna's grief deters him from his duty of fighting against the Kauravas, Shri Krishna consoles him. He advises him not to grieve for the Kauravas and fight against them. They are the ones who have done injustice to the Pandavas. Arjuna still remains grief-stricken. He fears that by killing the Kauravas he would kill his own relatives even though they had done injustice to the Pandavas. Then Krishna explains that he must not grieve for the Kauravas as ultimately they are bound to perish, because all who are born must die ultimately. In that process of consoling and advising Arjuna to fight so as to perform his duty, Krishna explains him the meaning of the Self. Krishna says:

अन्तवन्त इमे देहा नित्यस्योक्ताः शरीरिणः।
अनाशिनोऽप्रमेयस्य तस्माद्युध्यस्व भारत।। १८ ।।

Of this indwelling Self—the ever changeless, the indestructible, the illimitable—these bodies are said to have an end. Fight, therefore, O descendent of Bharata."[19]

"Krishna goes on enlightening Arjuna and remarks that 'he who takes the Self to be the slayer or takes it to be the slain, is ignorant, for it neither does slay nor is it slain'. A similar view of the Self is also contained in the *Kath Upnishad*.* Let me present in Sanskrit the subsequent Sloka (verse) from the Gita which further clarifies the meaning of the Self.

न जायते म्रियते वा कदाचिन्नायं भूत्वा भविता वा न भूयः।
अजो नित्यः शाश्वतोऽयं पुराणो, न हन्यते हन्यमाने शरीरे ।। २०।।

The verse explains that the Self is never born, nor does It die. It is not that, not having been, It again comes into being. (Or according to another view: It is not that having been, It again ceases to be.) This is unborn, eternal, changeless, ever-Itself. It is not killed when the body is killed.[20]

---

* Kath Upnishad, Chapter I ii, pp. 19–20.

Arjuna is still grief-stricken and is not prepared to fight the Kauravas. Obviously he is confused, mainly due to his ignorance (*Maya*). Knowing Arjuna's grief-stricken state, Krishna goes on consoling him. He remarks that if he knows that the Self is indestructible, changeless, immutable and without birth, he (Arjuna) is neither going to slay nor become the cause to slay anyone. Krishna continues consoling Arjuna and remarks: **This (Self) is said to be unmanifested, unthinkable and unchangeable. Therefore, knowing this (Self) to be such, he should not mourn.**[21]

Almost more than 2400 years back from now, when the Vedanta thought stream was in vogue in India, Krishna could not escape being influenced by it.

Thus, the *Bhagvad Gita* unfolds again and again the same thought process. The Gita's Self is, therefore, similar to that of the Advaita Vedanta.

Stream of Successive States

Chronologically, Buddha does not appear immediately after the Vedantic tradition. But we are considering the Buddhist point of view first, because, not only Buddha presented an unusual explanation towards the meaning of the soul, his disciples' and the monks' discussions are also quite fascinating and, therefore, note-worthy. Most of Buddhist traditions contain that the soul is non-existent. The explanation goes like this:

> *None is exempt from the law of change which is universal. It is believed that man possesses an abiding substance called the soul (atman), which, persists through changes that overcome the body. The soul exists before birth and after death and migrates from one body to another.*

Buddha consistently denies the existence of a soul with his theories of conditioned existence and universal change. Although Buddha does not accept the continuity of an identical substance in man, he does not deny the continuity of the stream of successive states that compose man's life. Buddha holds that life is an unbroken series of states. Each of these states depends on the condition just preceding and then giving rise to the succeeding state. In this manner the continuity of life series is based on a casual connection running through the different states.[22]

A beautiful example is presented by the Buddhists to explain this continuity. When a lamp burns throughout the night, the flame of each moment is dependent on its own conditions, and different from that of another moment that is dependent on other conditions. Yet there is an unbroken succession of different flames. As from one flame another may be lighted, though the two are different, they are surely connected casually. Similarly, Buddha holds that the end-state of this life may cause the beginning of the next life. Rebirth is, therefore, not transmigration, that is, migration of the soul into another body. Next the body is the causation of the next life by the present.[23]

Since the soul is defined as an unbroken stream of consciousness, memory becomes explicable even without a soul. Buddha, therefore, repeatedly emphasizes to his disciples to give up the false view about the Self. Buddha points out the people who suffer from the illusion of the self (soul), do not know its nature clearly. Still they strongly protest that they love the soul and they want to make the soul happy by obtaining salvation. It is just like building a stair-case for mounting a palace that never existed or seen.[24]

The Buddhists conceive that a person is only a conventional name for a collection of different constituents. These constituents are, the material body (*kaya*), the immaterial mind (*Manas or chitta*), the formless consciousness (*Vijnana*), just as a chariot is a collection of wheels, axles, shafts, etc. The existence of a person depends on this collection and it dissolves when the collection breaks up. The soul or the ego denotes nothing than this collection.[25]

The example of the chariot defining the doctrine of non-self comes from the account of the conversation between the Greek king Milinda and the Buddhist sage Nagasena. The sage explains to the Greek king that as the word chariot is merely a symbol for the parts 'assembled' or placed together in a particular way, in the same manner, the word 'self' also is only a label for the *aggregate* of certain physical and psychical factors. According to Buddhism, this *aggregate* does not continue the same for even two moments. It is constantly changing which is very well illustrated by the conceptions of 'the stream of water' and the 'self-consuming flame'. The latter being particularly appropriate in respect of the Self in that it is also suffering through its tormenting heat.[26]

In our search to know the 'Meaning of the Self' let us quote a few discourses held between the Buddhist monks and the masters in China and Japan.

Sekito (700–790) was one of the greatest figures in Buddhism of the T'ang dynasty. A monk called Shiri once asked him, "What is that which makes up this Self?" To this the master answered as a counter-question, "What do you want from me?"

The monk said, "If I do not ask you, where can I get the solution?"

"Did you ever lose it?" concluded the master.

Similarly, once Bunsui of Hoji monastery in Kinryo gave the following discourse to his monks: "O monks, you have been here for some time, the winter session is over and the summer has come. Have you had an insight into your Self, or not? If you have, let me be your witness, so that you will have a right view and not be led by wrong views."

Then a monk came forward and asked, "What is my Self?"

The master answered, "What a fine specimen of manhood with a pair of bright eyes!"[27]

I quote other discourses that took place in the monasteries. When one of the monks asked the master Yentoku of Yentsu, "What is my Self?", the master replied, "What makes you specially ask this question?"

Similarly, when a monk asked the master Ki of Unryu, "What is my Self?", the master replied: "It is like you and me?"

When the monk asked another question, "In this case there is no duality?"

The master replied, "18,000 miles off!"

At another occasion when a monk asked Yo of Kori monastery, "When I lack clear insight into my own Self, what shall I do?"

The master answered, "No clear insight!"

At this the monk said, "Why not?" Then the master Yo answered beautifully, "Don't you know that it's one's own business?"[28]

The answers given by the Buddhist masters to explain the meaning of the Self are sometimes subtle and sometimes quite lucid. The fact is that the answers require certain insight to know what constitutes the Self. It is difficult to understand it merely by thinking over intellectually.

Buddhist philosophy is built upon the most fundamental, pre-rationalistic *prajana*-intuition. When this is reached, such problems as the Self, Ultimate Reality, the Buddha-dharma, the Tao, the Source, the Mind, etc., are all solved.

After the Vedic traditions, Buddhist discourses are the great sources of knowledge to answer various questions relating to the Self, source of life, ultimate reality, or salvation. Once the master asked a monk, "Where do you come from?"

The monk answered, "I come from a monastery on the Western side of the river where Kwannon is enshrined."

The master said, "Did you see Kwannon?" The monk answered, "Yes, I did." At this the master inquired again, "Did you see it on the right side or the left side?"

The monk replied, "When seeing, there is neither right nor left."

In a *monoto* (discourse) like this, one can readily see that the question that issued is not Kwannon, which is used simply as the symbol for the Self, or the Tao, or Ultimate Reality, and the seeing of it means *prajana*-intuition. There is no differentiation in it of right and left; it is complete in itself; it is a unity itself; it is "pure" seeing. The monk apparently understood what *prajana*-intuition was, and this form of question on the part of the master is known as a "trial" question.[29]

A few more examples of master-monk discourses may highlight how the master, in order to provide right understanding, would answer difficult questions which involved the *prajana*-intuition.

Once a monk asked Kyoyu of Hoju monastery, "What is the ultimate principle of Buddhism?"

The master looked at him for a moment and replied, "Come nearer."

The monk moved forward, and the master said, "Do you understand?"

The monk said, "I do not master."

The master remarked, "It is like a flash of lightning, and it went eons ago."

Sometimes the masters replied questions in such a manner that their answers wouldn't be easily perceptible. For example, when a monk asked Soton of Dairin monastery, "How do we discourse on the highest truth of Buddhist philosophy?" To this the master replied, "Few hear it." The monk later came to Soton and inquired, "What did that mean?" Soton said, "When you have finished removing Mt. Sekiji, I will tell you."[30]

The masters were generally off the track of "logic", and would sometimes indulge in making fun of one another. They were often witty and sportive too. As they implied **prajana*-intuition to reach the truth, they naturally avoided getting into a philosophical discussion involving abstract ideas.** As a result they were partial to figures, imageries and facts of daily experience. At times they would say, "I don't know?" and they summed up the entire discourse. That means they did not want to indulge with the abstract questions further. Perhaps it was also in line with the Buddhist tradition.

Jiva is a Conscious Substance

The Jainas hold an important position among the ancient Indian philosophers. They define *jiva* (soul) or *atman* as a conscious substance. *Atman* (Self) in this world is known as *jiva*. It has vital physical, mental and sensuous powers. In its pure condition, *jiva* has *Nirvikalpa* (pure knowledge) and *Saviklpa Jnana* (vision of knowledge). The Jainas believe in the theory of previous life. Therefore, they believe that due to the effect of Karma (deeds accomplished in the previous and this life), *jiva* is yoked with various kinds of desires and with *Pudgala* (matter). The Jainas hold that *jiva* has different attributes. It is self-illuminated and illuminates other things also. It is a matter of interest that though Buddha and Jaina philosophies developed almost side by side, there is a great diversity in their approaches

* Prajana the fundamental neotic principle whereby a synthetic apprehension of the whole becomes possible.

** The masters frequently made such factually impossible statements. The idea is to make the questioners, that is all objectively minded people, reverse their way of thinking. Ultimately, this means to re-examine our ordinary "logical" way of reasoning.

towards the meaning of *jiva*. Rather Jainas seem to be more clear in conceiving the qualities of *jiva*. The Buddhist monks do not seem to be much concerned about it. To Jainas *jiva* is eternal and pervades the whole body. It enjoys the fruits of actions and tends to go upwards. *Karma* enters into it due to eternal ignorance and binds it in shackles. The fettered *jiva* is conscious. Possessed of the qualities of flexibility and resilience, it assumes the form of the body it enters. The *jiva* does not envelop the body but it can enter into matter. Similarly, one *jiva* can enter into another *jiva*. The *jiva* has no form and is, therefore, not the object of eyes. Its existence is determined by self-experience. In the released state it attains right knowledge. The *jiva* has various modes (body). It is ever characterized by birth, destruction and eternity. This is due to the effect of time. The *jiva* inherently possesses infinite perception, infinite knowledge and infinite power. Its manifestation is blocked by the clock of actions.

The Jainas believe that the *jiva* is of two kinds, *Baddha* (bound) *Mukta* (free). The former is further subdivided into categories, viz., *jangamaand sthavara*. The *sthavara jivas* possess only one sense organ, that is, either earth, water, fire, or the vegetable world. The *jivas* possessing more than one-sense organs are known as *trs*. Human beings, birds, animals, gods and devils are included in the category of *trs jivas*. These *jivas* have five sense organs. They have different names, which are determined by the kinds of bodies they possess. The *jivas* like stones, assume earthly bodies, etc.[31]

Jaina philosophy contends that there are proofs of the existence of the soul. These proofs are of two kinds, viz., direct and indirect. Jainas refute the Charvakas' views pertaining to the existence of the soul for they believe that consciousness is the finest element in the matter (body), and the soul as such is no separate entity. The Jainas consider Charvakas' view of soul as skeptical. They contend that with the attributes of qualities of soul, we directly realize the existence of soul. The perception of attributes tantamount to the perception of the substance. For example, if one feels that one is happy then the feeling of happiness enables one to have a direct realization of the existence of soul. Similarly, the existence of different attributes like sorrow, memory, thought, doubt and knowledge, leads to the direct realization of the possessor of these attributes, i.e. soul.[32] The Jainas also consider some indirect proofs of the existence of the soul. These are,

(i) One can move the body according to one's will. So there must be its mover, the soul.

(ii) The sense organs such as eyes, ears, etc., are the various instruments of knowledge. Without a coordinator, knowledge cannot be gathered through these sense-organs. The soul is the required coordinator.

(iii) Besides the material cause, an efficient cause is also required for the production of inanimate objects, that is, a glass, a jar or a piece of cloth. The body also cannot come into existence without an efficient cause. The soul is the efficient cause of the existence of the body.[33]

The Jainas analogy in respect of the soul's existence seems to be quite convincing. The characteristics attributed to the soul were not so clearly conceived by the Buddhists. Descartes is one of the foremost philosophers in the Western world, who tried to prove his own existence by expressing his famous sentence *Cogito ergo sum* (I think so I exist). Thus, he provided proofs for the soul's existence. The rest talked about the soul but they did not say much about its attributes. In the East, besides the Indian philosophers, there are Chinese thinkers, who have a highly developed philosophical system. The Chinese, from the beginning, had 2 complementary aspects of thought known as Confucianism and Taoism. They were practical people. They possessed a highly developed social consciousness. So they were concerned in one way, with life in society, with human relations, moral values and government. This, however, is only one aspect of their thought. Complementary to it is the mystical side of their character. It demanded that the highest aim of philosophy should be to transcend the world of society and everyday life and to reach a higher plane of consciousness. This is the way of the sage, the ideal of the enlightened person who has always tried to achieve mystical union with the universe.

A Chinese sage, however, does not dwell totally on this high spiritual plane. He is quite concerned with worldly affairs. He unifies in him the two complementary sides of human nature, that is, intuitive wisdom and practical knowledge, contemplation and social action, which the Chinese have associated with the images of the sage and of the king.[34] Therefore, they are not concerned with definitions and identification of the characteristics.

In our search for the meaning of Self, we continue our quest with 2 modern Indian philosophers—Acharya Rajneesh and Jiddu Kirshnamurti. With their distinguished power of eloquence and reasoning, they have attained a respectable position in the philosophical world. We take Rajneesh first.

Self as the Being

Acharya Rajneesh, more commonly known as Bhagwan Rajneesh, remained overcast on the philosophic horizon of the world for a good number of years. Before he was made to leave Rajneeshpuram (1985), which he had built in Oregon in the United States, he had a good number of rich disciples. They joined him with free will to seek knowledge, tranquillity and freedom. After he became popular he conducted big audiences. Naturally he used to have question and answer hours, during which he would respond to the queries of his inquisitive disciples and visitors. In one of those sessions when Rajneesh was analyzing the term 'self respect', someone asked him, "What is the place of surrender in your religion?" In that context Rajneesh explained the meaning of the Self too. He said:

> *The word self-respect may create doubts in your mind because self-respect seems to mean again the ego. It is not so. You have to understand both words "Self" and "respect"; both are significant. He continued, Self is that which you are born with. Ego is that which you accumulate. Ego is your achievement. Self is a gift of existence to you. You have not done anything to earn it, you have not achieved it; hence nobody can take it away from you. That is impossible because it is your nature, your very being.*[35]

Rajneesh goes on to explain the meaning of the Self. He contends that all the religions teach surrender, but ego must not be surrendered. It should be seen. It should be understood through and through. Only then the Self can be known. He explains that the meaning of respect is re-spect, which means to look again and go deep into one's own existence. It is the only way to find the place where from one started losing oneself. This is how one can know one's own self. Thus, Rajneesh describes the Self as one's own existence that is devoid of ego, and to know or understand the Self one need not surrender ego but see it thoroughly.

At another occasion when Rajneesh was answering questions, "Who is God?" and "Who created the world?", He said:

> *A mature mind has only one question. Not even two, just a single question: Who am I? And that too you have not to ask verbally, you have just to be in that state of questioning. You are not to repeat, 'Who am I?' You have just to be there, watching, looking: not verbally asking, but existentially asking.*[36]

Thus, Rajneesh without describing the Self's characteristics or going into further details about it, explains its meaning. He lets it open for us to reckon, "What does the Self mean?" In his process of defining the Self, he seems to be following Buddhist masters' tradition and manner. Rajneesh was a great intellectual who could analyze things to the extent of great clarity. He knew how difficult it would be to deal directly with the meaning of the Self. Therefore, the procedure he adopts is interesting, self explanatory, and awakening as well. Let us now examine the Self from Jiddu Krishnamurti's point of view.

Self as an Entity

In his search for the meaning of the Self and human freedom, Krishnamurti provides a new line of thought. Before explaining its meaning directly, he explains to us the circumstances that are detrimental in finding out the correct meaning of the Self. Until one is totally free from those circumstances, confusion and turmoil, one cannot possess the knowledge of its own self. He believes that it is only the confusion of the human mind, which is inherent in its habitual modes of thought, that inhibits the experience of true freedom. As the mind is habitually preoccupied, consequently it has grown insensitive to the whole movement and process of life in man and nature. The fundamental problems for the human being, says Krishnamurti, is the question of man's freedom from his little corner. That little corner is ourselves. That little corner is our own shoddy little mind as it is fragmented and, therefore, incapable of being sensitive to the whole. If we really desire to expand the mind and break its confinement from "the little corners', we need to liberate it from a kind of psychological bondage. It would lead us to know the Self and help us understand the wholeness of life.[37]

On one occasion when Krishnamurti was addressing some visitors who had come to listen to him, he explained the difference between the meaning of an individual and a human being. He said:

> *And what is yourself, the individual you? I think there is a difference between the human being and an individual...The individual is the little conditioned, miserable, frustrated entity, satisfied with his little gods and his little traditions, whereas a human being is concerned with the total welfare, the total misery and total confusion of the world.*[38]

Krishnamurti holds that as the individual is conditioned, he has been influenced by religion, tradition and customs for years. So he cannot see through the truth that is something living, moving and has no resting place. It can neither be found in a temple, nor in a mosque, a church and to which no religion, no teacher, no philosopher—nobody can lead us to. In pursuit of truth one has to leave behind all sorts of conditioning. Only then one will be able to see the living thing—what one actually is. Therefore, the Self is only an entity. It could be perceived and known clearly if it is devoid of all kinds of conditioning, including, religion, tradition, words and even fear. When the Self is free from all that, it is most natural, real and true. "Then you will see that living thing what you actually are—your anger, your brutality, your violence, your despair, the agony and sorrow you live in. In the understanding of all this is the truth,..."[39]

Krishnamurti defines the meaning of the Self more comprehensively in his book, *The First and Last Freedom.* This seems to be based on his experience as a human being. He narrates:

Do you know what we mean by the Self? By that, I mean the idea, the memory, the conclusion, the experience, the various forms of nameable and unnameable intentions, the conscious endeavour to be or not to be, the accumulated memory of the unconscious, the racial, the group, the individual, the clan, and the whole of it all, whether it is projected outwardly in action or projected spiritually as virtue; the striving after all this is the Self. In it is included the competition, the desire to be. The whole process of that is the Self.[40]

Krishnamurti believes that in understanding the meaning of the Self, one needs to know the importance of the experience that strengthens the Self. Do we not have experiences all the time? We translate those experiences or impressions and react or act according to them. There is a constant interplay between what is seen objectively and our reactions to it which interplay between the conscious and the memories of the unconscious. According to our memories, we react to whatever we see or feel, know or believe, experience is taking place. Krishnamurti continues elaborating its meaning. He states that desires play some role in the projection of the Self. One desires to be projected or desires to have a master or a guru, a teacher or a God. When one projects a desire, it takes a form, to which one gives a name, e.g., "I have met the Master", etc. There could be another desire, like, "I want to understand what is truth. It is my longing, which is followed by a projection and consequently experience takes place." That experience provides strength to the Self. Thus the Self becomes one with the experience. Then one says, "I know it" or "I know that God exists or does not exist." Therefore, experience is always strengthening the 'Me'. As a result of that, one gets strength of character, strength of knowledge, of belief, which one constantly displays through speech or behaviour. "In that process of experience, reaction and projection, the Self is isolated or is always involved with all the above. Can we go to the root of it and understand the process which would enable us to know the Self?"[41]

Krishnamurti holds that various forms of discipline, beliefs or knowledge only strengthen the Self. Is it then possible to dissolve the

Self? Perhaps yes, is the answer from Krishnamurti. He believes that those who are integrally intelligent only they can dissolve the Self. Thus, according to Krishnamurti, understanding of the Self requires a great deal of intelligence, great deal of watchfulness, alertness in watching ceaselessly, so that it does not slip away.

Krishnamurti elucidates the issue, 'Whether the Self can be dissolved!' He comments that when mind seeks a timeless spiritual state in order to destroy the Self, it goes into another form of experience. It leads to strengthening 'Me'. For example, when one believes that there is truth, God or immortality, it again involves the process of strengthening the Self. Then the Self projects according to one's own beliefs, which involves experience. This does not lead to destroy the Self. If one observes inwardly, one would find that the same action goes on and on and the same 'Me' functions at different levels with different labels and different names. [42]

Then what should be done to dissolve the Self that has been created by the whole process of experience, involving belief, knowledge, identification, etc.? The only way to destroy it, says Krishnamurti, is to observe it, see it that the mind is not moving in a circle, in a cage of its own. When one comes to that point—not ideologically, or through projected experience, he is free from conditioning. When one's mind is actually in that state of observation, it becomes completely still and has no power to create. Then there is creation that is not a common process already known. Thus, step by step, Krishnamurti explains the meaning of the Self. One can know the Self not by having the accumulated experience or possessing beliefs or identification, but by keeping the mind detached from the self-creation. That kind of creation is the result of the past experience and constant conditioning. Krishnamurti contends that the only way to know the Self is to keep the mind alert, watchful and aware of its movements. Then the mind is in a state of silence by becoming a dispassionate observer. It becomes free.

Retrospection

We are almost at the close of our discussion on the meaning of the Self. We started with the Western thinkers—first with Socrates. He defined soul as the most truly a man's self, that is the normal waking personality and the seat of character and intelligence. His disciple, Plato, described it as a *distinct immaterial essence or being, imprisoned in the body*. Its nature has not much to do with the earthly as its home and destiny are the world of ideas. Plato further classifies soul having three parts or functions that correspond with reason, will and feeling. Out of them 'reason' is the 'divine' part, while the latter two are close to the physical body and, therefore, are not immortal.

Aristotle recognizes soul quite in line with Plato, but he considers it having a close relation to the body also. He views soul *as the very perfection of the body*. David Hume bluntly remarks that we have no experience of any such thing as a soul at all. There is no evidence for its existence. He thinks that our experience provides us lots of impressions or perceptions, ideas or memory images, and *soul is simply a collection of these impressions and ideas*. Emmanuel Kant does not like to indulge himself in defining its meaning. He remarks that Hume is right that *soul or self is revealed through experience*, which provides impressions and memory images. Therefore, the knowledge of the Self was difficult. Still, Kant has no doubt at all as to the fact of there being a Self, but what that Self is, is beyond human knowledge.

William Mc Dougall, describing the philosophy of mind, use the terms like soul, ego, or Self for mind and considers it as *a unitary and distinct psychic being. It cannot be identified with body*. In the history of philosophy, mind has been identified in different ways. Those views or theories are classified under 5 heads. They are:

1. Subjective theory of Descartes, who holds that mind or soul is a separate and independent entity.
2. The second theory (epiphenomenalistic) conceives mind as the by-product of the body, and the soul perishes with the body.
3. The third theory, advocated by Hume, denies a subjective mind and holds that 'mind' is simply a succession of experiences or mental states.
4. The fourth is the functional view propounded by Aristotle. According to that, mind is an adaptive instrument, developed in the long course of evolution.
5. The fifth is the behaviouristic theory which holds that mind is simply the behaviour of certain organism.

The above theories converse towards definite results. One of these is the Freudian emphasis on vital impulses that often drive us on, apparently, with some conscious purpose. The next one is

Warren's view, who concludes that the adaptive behaviour has a subjective side, which we call consciousness or experience. There is another belief emphasized by Plato who contends that there is a peculiar unitary personal character of the Self. Finally Aristotle's views according to which, the mind is the perfection and fruition of the body. Aristotelian views in respect of the soul are getting more serious attention which is evident in movements such as the Gestalt theory.

Patrick and some other thinkers hold that consciousness is not synonymous to mind, though it has often been done in the past. It may be better to say that consciousness accompanies all mental states and processes. But that may also be questioned. Freudians have developed a widely accepted theory of mind, in which unconscious mental elements play important parts. Thus, philosophers have accepted widely that mind and consciousness are not the same. Bertrand Russell holds that consciousness is not an essence of life. It is not also a kind of substance out of which mind is made. We cannot think of it as an entity or quality of being itself, thinks William James. Then what is consciousness?

Warren explains both, mind and consciousness quite lucidly. He states, 'When adaptive behaviour is witnessed in others, we call it mind, but when it is experienced in ourselves, it is called consciousness. In fact, conscious phenomena are merely mental phenomena as they appear subjectively in our experience. **Consciousness is thus a kind of privacy—an intimate, inner, serious aspect of mental life which is not completely revealed to the observation of others'.** Being a kind of inner and intimate aspect of mental life, it cannot be taken as the whole mind or soul. But it is surely a distinct feature of mind or soul. Thus, mind and consciousness are two different things.

The Vedantics contend that the Self is quite akin to that of the Self what Sankhya-Yoga holds. They conceive it as extraneous to the apparatus (body), that in the same way helps its manifestation. Then ultimately, it goes back to the same source, viz., Brahman or Spirit. In the *Bhagwad Gita*, Shri Krishna conceives that the Self is never born nor it dies. It is changeless, eternal and never ceases to be. It is not destructible, nor it can be slain. It cannot be a slayer too. The *Kath Upnishad* contains similar views about the soul.

According to most Buddhist traditions the soul is non-existent. Buddha believed that in man there is an abiding substance called the soul (*atman*), which persists through changes that overcome the body, exists before birth and after death, and migrates from one body to another. The Buddhists elucidate this phenomenon through the example of a burning lamp which each moment is not the same and with it another lamp can be lighted. Thus, soul is an unbroken stream of consciousness. The Jainas conceive *java* or *atman* (soul) as a conscious substance. Atman in this world is known as *jiva*. It has vital and physical, mental and sensuous powers. The Jainas believe in the previous life and due to the effect of *karma, jiva* is yoked with *pudgala* (matter) on account of its various kinds of desires. According to the Jainas the *jiva* has different attributes. It is self-illuminated and illuminates other things too. The *jiva* has no form and, therefore, cannot be seen by eyes. Its existence is determined by self-experience and when it is in the realized state, it attains right knowledge.

The Jainas believe that there are direct and indirect proofs of the existence of the soul. They contend that with the immediate knowledge of its attributes, the soul can be directly realized. For example, the feeling of happiness is a direct realization of its existence. Similarly, when one experiences sorrow, thought, doubt and knowledge, it leads to the direct knowledge of these attributes or soul. The indirect proofs of its existence are the movements of the body which, are done by its mover, the soul. The sense organs like eyes, ears, etc. are the instruments of knowledge, but without a coordinator knowledge cannot be gathered through the sense organs, and without the efficient cause, which is the soul. The body cannot come into existence without the soul. These direct and indirect proofs of soul's existence also formulate its definition. Rajneesh defines the Self as man's existence with which he is born. In order to know the Self, man has to see and understand his ego and look into his own self. He needs not to surrender his ego but see it through and through; only then he would know his own real Self.

Jiddu Krishnamurti presents a new line of thought before us in quest of understanding the meaning of the Self. In order to understand the Self, one would require to break the mind's confinement from the 'little corners' that create psychological bondage to it. Only then one can know the Self and understand the wholeness of life. Krishnamurti contends that if one wants to know the truth, one must leave behind all kind of conditioning. Then one would be able to see the living thing—what one actually is. Perhaps among all the modern thinkers, Krishnamurti seems to be quite pragmatic in elucidating the meaning of the Self. He reflects upon all those factors too that stand as impediments to the knowledge of the Self. He argues that conditioning is created either by tradition, word, religion, fear or repeatedly hammered thoughts. When the conditioning is removed, the Self illuminates in its reality. Then this living thing often comprised with (one's) anger, brutality, despair, violence, agony and sorrow, would be understood actually. In knowing all that is the Truth, is to know the real Self. Thus, Krishnamurti recognizes the modes of life as part of the Self or Self itself. Like David Hume, Krishnamurti also contends that experience plays a great role in man's understanding and knowing. Krishnamurti adds that experience and desire both, play a great role in the formation of conditioning. When one experiences or desires something, reaction takes place as a result of the projection of the desire. It leads to some kind of experience too. Thus, in that process of experience, reaction and projection, the real Self is lost or it gets conditioned. Therefore, to know the Self, one has to go to the root of it and dissolve the Self away from all the experience, reactions and projections that are the basis of all conditioning. Thus, to conceive the pure form of the Self, one needs to be integrally intelligent, which requires a great deal of watchfulness and alertness. If one can become a dispassionate observer and an on looker, and can watch ceaselessly, one can gradually attain the silence of mind. Then one will be in a state of mind to know the Self.

Why Know the Self!

After all that discussion about 'what is the meaning of the Self?', a thought comes to my mind, 'Whether there is any need to understand the meaning of the Self!' My immediate response to it would be that it is surely imperative to know the nature of the Self. When a person dies and his conscious Self and the living body are gone, what remains behind is the dead stuff. No one loves it, neither preserves it for future (except the mummies of Egypt that were preserved for certain reasons). Therefore, the spirit or the Self is the most precious thing in person. It is the life force, comprised with thinking, feeling as well as reasoning. One cannot live without the activities such as feeling, thinking and reasoning as they make him move and help fulfilling his goals. This is perhaps one reason that he needs to know about the Self—his own Self.

Besides, it is also important for him to know, 'What is the real mission of his life?' Is it meant to quench the thirst of his sensuous desires or it has some higher purpose to live? What acts or thoughts make him temporarily happy and what activities bring him lasting happiness? These are some of the important aspects of human life that are directly connected with the soul. The truth is, that as a consequence to man's pious or impious activities or thoughts, the soul ultimately reacts. It can be confirmed from certain events that happen during man's life. For example, when someone helps a needy or a sick person, the kind of happiness he experiences is unique. Likewise, a dying person in his last statement, even if he has been a hardcore culprit, invariably tells the truth. It is also quite likely that a person during his lifetime, may discover that certain activities bring him remorse or happiness. To cultivate this kind of understanding he needs to develop a habit of good thinking. It was the reason that the great Buddha among his eight-fold paths, included 'right mindfulness'. He thought that it would constantly keep person in touch with good. So it is quite imperative to know the meaning of one's own Self as the Self is implicit with the divine qualities and, therefore, it goes on directing him to act rightly.

Every time when a person reacts emotionally, his interests, desires, likes and dislikes are involved with those reactions. He often passes judgments on his own or others' actions by involving his own ego without trying to see things from a distance. Only if he can understand the causes of his reactions projected by self-interests, it would become easier for him to take decisions correctly and his life would have become much happier. In this way it is quite important that a person knows himself thoroughly and intimately. Without it he would never understand his reactions and know his inadequacies or strength. The truth is that most people do not have any desire to peep into themselves. Therefore, they never know their own Self. It became clear to me when I interviewed hundreds of people in India and abroad. The fact is that hardly a handful of them answered my question(s) relating to the Self. Since my own knowledge about it was not very adequate, I had two options to know more about it. One by reading as much as I could, and the other was to talk to the educated people from all walks of life. A small number of people who really willingly responded to my questions and who believed to have understood the meaning of the Self, reported that:

Soul or Self is the best part of an individual's consciousness—a kind of touchstone to judge our actions by which when approved, give us the greatest pleasure and when disapproved, leave a sense of guilt and bitter sadness. Everyone, including a hard-core criminal, has a soul—it is muted or outspoken, depends largely on one's desire to listen to it. Therefore, our actions are in direct correspondence with soul's guidance.

Besides, some also added that 'The first reaction or impulse to an action is the voice of soul, therefore, good.' It gives way when ignored due to other impulses. Most people who tried to respond to my question, couldn't provide a clear and objective answer to it. They were not academically inadequate, but perhaps they did not try to transcend their religious and cultural prejudices. I, therefore, strongly felt to know more about the nature of the Self and to discover a comprehensive meaning of it. Thus, as a consequence to my findings this chapter has been prepared. Although it does not contain any pin-pointed definition of the Self, it does provide views of the ancient and the most modern thinkers about it, telling us what the Self really is.

Perhaps, the basic difficulty in conceiving the meaning of the Self crops up, when we do not try to dislodge from us our longings and desires relating to the material world. Some take this world to be totally illusory as it is impermanent, while others conceive it existing really, even though it is constantly changing. Therefore, it becomes necessary to understand the concept of dualism, as without conceiving it properly, the knowledge of the Self would perhaps remain inadequate.

References

1. Cora Mason, Socrates: *The Man Who Dared to Ask*, pp. 8–11.
2. Plato, *The Dialogue of Plato : Apology*, (trans.), Vol. II, p. 125.
3. S. Radhakrishnan, *History of Philosophy: Eastern and Western*, (Ed), p. 51.
4. Plato, *Apology*, pp. 123–124.
5. Julian Marian, *History of Philosophy*, p. 47.
6. G.T.W. Patric, *Introduction to Philosophy*, pp. 241–242.
7. L.R. Loomis, *Aristotle : Man in the Universe*, pp. 85–86.
8. Loomis, *Aristotle : Man in the Universe*, pp. 93–94.
9. Marian, *History of Philosophy*, pp. 78–79.
10. David Hume, *Treatise on Human Nature*, Book I, Part iv, p. 6.
11. Hume, *Treatise on Human Nature*, Book I, Part iv, p. 6.
12. Patric, *Introduction to Philosophy*, pp. 248–250.
13. Patric, *Introduction to Philosophy*, pp. 263–264.
14. Patric, *Introduction to Philosophy*, p. 284.
15. William James, "Does Consciousness Exist?", *Journal of Philosophy, Psychology, Science and Maths*, Vol. I, pp. 447–91.
16. Patric, *Introduction to Philosophy*, p. 285.
17. S. Alexander and Wendell T. Bush, "An Empirical Definition Consciousness," *Journal of Philosophy , Psychology, Science and Maths*, Vol. II, p. 561.
18. M. Hiriyanna, *Outlines of Indian Philosophy*, pp. 342–344.
19. Swami Swarupananda, *Shrimad Bhagwad Gita*, Verse 18, p. 39.
20. Swarupananda, *Bhagwad Gita*, Verse 20, p. 40.
21. Swarupananda, *Bhagwad Gita*, p. 43.
22. H.C. Warren, *Buddhism in Translation*, p. 233.
23. Warren, *Buddhism in Translation*, p. 234 f.
24. S.C. Chatterjee & D. Dutta, *An Introduction to Indian Philosophy*, p. 140.
25. Rhy Davids, *Dialogues of Buddha*, (Eng. trans.) pp. 259–261.
26. Hiriyanna, *Essentials of Indian Philosophy*, pp. 140–141.
27. *Records of the Translations of the Transmission of the Lamp*, (RTL) pp. xxv 77b.
28. RTL, pp. xxv, 86 b; & RTL, pp. xxii, 45 b.
29. G.E. Moore, *Lectures on Philosophy*, pp. 36–37.
30. RTL, pp. xxvi, 85 b.
31. R.N. Sharma, *Indian Philosophy*, pp. 122–123.
32. R.N. Sharma, *Indian Philosophy*, pp. 123–124.
33. R.N. Sharma, *Indian Philosophy*, p. 124.
34. Fritjof Capra, *The Tao of Physics*, pp. 91–92.

35. Bhagwan Shree Rajneesh, *Rajneesh Bible*, Vol. II, pp. 816-817.
36. Rajneesh, *The Rajneesh Bible*, Vol. III, pp. 210–211.
37. Stuart Holroyd, *Quest of the Quiet Mind*, p. 45.
38. Jiddu Krishnamurti, *Freedom From the Known*, pp. 12–13.
39. Krishnamurti, *Freedom From the Known*, p. 15.
40. Krishnamurti, *Freedom From the Known*, p. 76.
41. Krishnamurti, *The First and Last Freedom*, p. 78.
42. Krishnamurti, *The First and Last Freedom, pp. 80–81.*

2

Concept of Duality

It seems quite important to discuss the concept of duality in view of our discussions in the preceding chapter. I, therefore, present the views of the philosophers, who, while trying to discover the true nature of the Self, also confided that there were two kinds of realities—matter and mind. Without discussing the relationship of matter with mind, our discussions on the knowledge of Self, may perhaps remain incomplete. This chapter, thus contains the views of the Western and the Eastern philosophers, who made great efforts in explaining the problem of dualism.

Western Dilemma

The Greek philosophers put great efforts in overcoming the sharp contrast between the views of Parmenides and Heraclitus. It was the 5th century BC. In order to reconcile the idea of the unchangeable Being propounded by Permenides and with that of eternal becoming of Heraclitus, they assumed that the Being is manifested in certain invariable substances. Mixture and separation of that give rise to the changes in the world, that perhaps, led to the concept of the atom, the smallest indivisible unit of matter. Democritus often expressed it in his discourses. The Greek philosophers, therefore, drew a clear line between matter and spirit, reckoning matter as being made of several "basic building blocks". These were purely passive and intrinsically dead particles moving in the void. They never explained the cause of their motion. The motion was often associated with external forces that were assumed to be of spiritual origin, being fundamentally different from matter.[1]

As the idea of a division between spirit and matter got a firm footing, philosophers turned their attention to the spiritual world rather than the material. Thus, the human soul and the problem of ethics took of paramount importance for them. It was impossible for Socrates to stay out of the influence of those ancient Greek thinkers. Thus, his search for finding out the nature of *truth, beauty* and *goodness* grew to the extent that he did not hesitate to sacrifice his own life to discover their meaning.

Socrates did not get much time for himself to do more than clarifying the doubts of the people and defining the nature of truth. But he laid down the foundation on which Plato made the structure of his philosophy. In that process of enlightening people, he developed a technique, known as Socratizing. He led people to conceive the answers of their own queries that they often put to him in quest of truth. Before Socrates, cosmology had been the chief topic of interest, but after him the central problem was to formulate a rule of life. Therefore, with him the 'practical use of reason' came by its rights. Socrates, during his short stay, stamped on philosophy a character that it has never lost. The main outline of Socrates' philosophy can be discovered through Platonic *Apology*. It tells us that some specific message from God was brought to his fellow men by his Master. The message was that 'it is the greatest business of life to practise the "care" or "tendencies" of the soul, to make one's soul as good as possible, and not to ruin one's life as most men do, by putting care for the body or for "possessions" before care for the soul'.*

The fundamental thought that is that the 'soul' is most truly a man's Self. From the beginning of the fourth century we find coming at last to mean what 'soul' means to us. It is reckoned as normal waking personality, the seat of character and intelligence, "that", as Socrates says to Plato, "in virtue of which we are called wise or foolish, good or bad".* We have already stated it that Socrates contended that our happiness or well-being depends directly on the goodness or badness of the soul. One cannot claim to possess happiness, strength, health or wealth unless one knows how to use these advantages rightly. If one uses them wrongly, they will only be so many means to misery. Therefore, the soul can hardly be separated from divinity. In establishing the absolute worth and dignity to the soul, Plato

* Encyclopedia Britannica, Vol. 20, p. 920.

in his beautiful dialogue, called the *Phaedo*, attempted to establish the truth of immortality of the soul upon philosophic grounds. In many passages relating to its immortality, he exalted the soul. He identified it with the vision of the absolute and as having kinship with God. Perhaps that could have been the reason to narrate the 'Simile of the Cave' in his *Republic*. In it he gives a account of the people belonging to the two worlds, the noumenal and the phenomenal. That is, the physical and that which can be known through the intellect. Through that 'Simile' he presented an idea that 'people live in ignorance until they are free from their fetters created by illusion.' It was certainly an alarming concept, to which Plato could hardly provide a very satisfactory explanation through his reasoning and discussions. Let us consider his views in that respect a little further.

Noumenal and Phenomenal

Plato presented primarily the idea of two kinds of worlds in the West. He conceived that 'there is a noumenal as well as phenomenal world. The soul itself has two divisions—both perceiving the world of material and form separately.' It became the starting point for both, Democritus and Plato. Both admitted that perception that was the product of a natural process, could be the knowledge of something only 'which arises and passes away as transitory product of the same natural process.' Plato thought that perception would not provide more than opinion. 'It provides what appears in and for human, not what *truly* or really is.'[2]

Both, Democritus and Plato were against the kind of knowledge sought from the senses. They thought that it was just an opinion. They acknowledged the reality of perception and transcended by accepting that "thought" was the true knowledge or the source of real knowledge. If the ideas (thought) are to be "something other" than the perceptible world, knowledge of them through conceptions cannot be found in the concept of perception. The ideas cannot be contained in it. With this kind of reasoning that clearly indicates that there are two kinds of worlds, the platonic doctrine of knowledge becomes much more rationalistic.

However, the concept of the *soul* or mind was itself a difficulty in dualism after Plato presented his doctrine of Ideas. For him "soul" was on one hand the living element, that which is moved to itself and moves other things. On the other hand, it is that which perceives, knows and wills. As a principle of life and motion, the soul belongs to the lower world of the Becoming. It remains in it when it perceives and directs its desires towards objects of the senses. The soul by its true knowledge of Ideas becomes particular in the higher reality of abiding Being. Therefore, it must be assigned a place *between the two worlds*—not the timeless, unchanged essence of Ideas, but a vitality that survives change; i.e., immortality.[3]

As a consequence of this intermediate position, the soul must bear in itself the qualities (traits) of both worlds. There must be in its essence something that corresponds to the world of perception. The former is the *rational nature,* the seat of knowledge and virtue that corresponds to it. In the latter, it is the irrational nature. Plato made further distinction of two elements—the nobler, that inclines towards the reason, and the lower, that resists it. The nobler possessed with the spirited will, the lower the sensuous desires. Thus, reason, spirit and appetite are the three forms of activity of the soul. The fettering of the soul to the body is at once a consequence and a punishment of the sensuous appetite; the immortal existence of the soul is beyond the two boundaries of the earthly life.[4]

We have already stated that philosophers have been trying to seek the meaning of a 'true being' since the time of Permenides. He believed that the true being does not reside in things, but outside of them in the Ideas. These are *metaphysical entities that cannot be true being of things*. They are that which authentically exists. The ideas are one, *changeless eternal,* they contain no admixture of non-being; they are not subject to motion or decay; they absolutely and unconditionally are.[5]

The being of things, that is a subordinate and defective being, is founded on the being of the Ideas in which the things share. Plato, thus, originates the division of reality into two worlds. He does not credit the world of things perceived by the senses. The world of the Ideas, that is true and full-being.[6]

Samkara's concept of Advaita is almost parallel to Platonic vision of the two worlds. The difference lies in their approaches and reasoning to know the nature of reality. Plato conceives the material world unreal as things are shadows of the Ideas. The world of 'forms' or Ideas, is the only real thing for him. For Samkara, it is

Maya or ignorance, that is the sole cause of illusion. The physical world (*Prakrit*) is only an appearance and therefore it is false or in Advaitic terminology, "other than real and unreal". Brahman is the ultimate reality and the primary cause of the world. We shall discuss Samkara, in this chapter, later on, when we have completed our discussion on the Western thinkers. Plato comes across a rather paradoxical situation while investigating the being of things. First, to know things for what they are and the things that are and are not (do not truly exist). Next to understand how it is possible for the things to come to be and cease to be—in general. Then, how they move or change without contradicting the traditional predicates of the Entity. How one would explain the oneness of the Entity compatible with the multiplicity of the things, etc. These were the situations or the questions that needed clear, satisfactory and convincing answers. When the things have no being, they cannot help to discover the being. How then one should seek them? When, according to Plato, true being resides in the Ideas, that are not directly accessible to one's consciousness, they are precisely not in the world. Nevertheless one knows them (ideas) in some way. They are with him and thus permit him as persons have seen to know the things.

Plato was quite aware of those paradoxes that were evolving out of his previous discussions. Therefore, to solve the problem he relates to a myth, which Socrates relates to Phaedrus on the bank of the river Ilissus. We have already narrated it in the first chapter of this book. The myth contains that the soul is compared to a chariot drawn by two winged horses, one a docile thorough-bred, the other an ungovernable steed (passions and sensual instincts). The charioteer (reason) strives to guide it properly. In a region above heaven the chariot travels through the world of Ideas, that the soul thus contemplates, although not without difficulty. Troubles arise in guiding the flight of the two horses, and the soul falls; the horses lose their wings and the soul becomes incarnated in a body. If the soul has seen the ideas, even though only briefly, this body will be human and not bestial. Plato believes that depending on the greater or lesser extent of the contemplation of the Ideas, souls are placed in a hierarchy of nine grades. They range from the philosophers down to the tyrant. The origin of person as such, is the fall of a soul that has come from heaven and has contemplated Ideas there. The incarnated person does not remember them.

Plato with greater emphasis explains that things are *shadows and Ideas*. Shadows are signs of things and they can make one aware of the existence of things. The mutilated stumps, that are remains of the former wings, when get agitated and long for regeneration, there is a feeling of restlessness like a painful itching. The virtue of wings consists in lifting heavy things upwards. They bear them through air to the place where the race of the gods reside. The contents of the said myth can be reduced in its essentials to the 'Simile of the Cave' of which a brief reference was made in the beginning of this chapter. Plato pictures that some persons have remained from their childhood in a cave. It has an opening in such a way that they cannot move or look in any direction than at the back of the cave. Outside the cave, behind the men's backs, there blazes the bright glow of a fire burning on a lofty place in the terrain. Between the fire and the chained men there is a road with a low wall along it. Down this road pass men carrying all sorts of objects and small statues that rise above the top of the wall. The chained men see the shadows of these things projected onto the back of the cave.

When the passers-by speak, it seems to the prisoners that those voices proceed from the shadows they see—their only reality. When one of the prisoners gets free from the chains, he views the real world outside. He sees the sky at night, the stars and the moon and at dawn, first the reflected image of the sun and finally after sometime he can look at the sun. Then he realizes that the world he lived before was unreal and contemptible. What is symbolized in this myth, is, that the cave is the world perceived by the senses, and its shadows are the things of the world of the senses. The world outside, is the true world, that is perceived by the mind or the world of Ideas. The objects of the outside world symbolize the Ideas. The sun symbolizes the Idea of the Good. Thus, Plato distinguishes two great regions of reality, the world of senses (of things) and the world of the mind (of Ideas).

The myth of the cave, narrated by Plato adds something to it. In concrete fashion, it symbolizes simultaneously the ontological structure of reality and meaning of philosophy. Thus, it introduces the fundamental oneness of those two worlds. The two great regions of reality are united into one reality by virtue of the role played by man, who comes face to face with both of them. The visible world and the world of the mind now appear related to two essential human potentialities: seeing and understanding. The man who is at first in the cave and then in the light, is one who gives a unity to the two worlds. The world as a whole is a double world integrated by man's passage from darkness to light. From another point of view, there is a second unifying link: the Good, the ontological basis of the being of both worlds.[7]

Soul as Realization of Body

Aristotle, in his search for reality, seems to differ from his predecessor and master, Plato. It goes to his credit that he systematized and organized the scientific knowledge of the past. He created the scheme that became the basis of the Western thought about the universe for almost 2000 years. He understood Plato to have held that 'universals' have objective existence. Plato really said so. He had said that 'the universals are incomparably more lasting, important and substantial than the individuals. 'Aristotle's is a matter-of-fact mind and, therefore, he sees the root of endless mysticism and scholarly nonsense in this Platonic "realism". So he attacks it with all vigour of a first potemic.'[8] He differs with Plato in many ways. His beliefs pertaining to human soul and God's perfection, are far more mature and valuable than his Master's. He boldly contends that the soul is the principle of life—the 'form' or realization of living body. In his opinion, the soul 'informs' or gives form to the matter of living things, giving it its 'corporal being' and making it a live body. Thus, it is not a question of the soul's being superimposed on the body but the body is a living body because it has a soul. With all these explanations, Aristotle clearly accepts that his belief in the reality of the soul is more paramount. He does not refute the reality of body, though it became a living body on account of the soul.

Worlds of Reality and Appearances

Plato and Aristotle are not the only philosophers who admit the existence of the world of reality. They accept somehow the world of appearances too. Their belief in the existence of the two worlds have been recognized by many philosophers in the Western world. However, their reasons of for accepting the world of reality and the world of appearances are not always the same as Plato's or even Aristotle's. Most outstanding of those philosophers is Emmanuel Kant. He is slightly apart from Plato and the others.

He admitted the dichotomy of the world of reality and the world of appearances for particular reasons. He, unlike Plato, held that the world of appearance is characterizable by *knowability par excellence,* but that the world of reality is *unknown* and *unknowable.* His doctrine of the unknowability of reality marks a departure from the metaphysics of Ultimate Reality belonging to the Platonic tradition. Kant left the door open for our access to it and held that the access lies in faith born of our moral consciousness. More important than it is Kant's admission of the dichotomy of the world of reality and the world of appearances.

Mind controls the Body

Before the birth of the modern science, in the 17th century, a new development took place in the field of philosophical thought. It led to an extreme formulation of the spirit/matter dualism. This formulation appeared in the philosophy of Rene Descartes. He based his view of nature on a fundamental division into two separate and independent realms: that of mind and matter. Descartes' philosophical views have exerted tremendous influence on the general Western way of thinking up to the modern times. His famous sentence *Cogito ergo sum,* "I think, therefore I exist" has led people throughout the world to think and to equate their identity with their mind, instead of with their total organism. As a result, most individuals would feel that they are aware of themselves as isolated egos existing "inside" their bodies. This notion not only created a feeling of division between mind and body but also gaves it (mind) the authority and task of controlling it. As a consequence, conflict between the conscious will and the involuntary instincts was quite apparent. Besides, Descartes thought that each individual seemed to have been split up further into a large number of compartments. According to his/her activities, talents, feelings, beliefs, etc., each individual engaged himself/herself in endless conflicts, creating continuous confusion in the philosophical world. With all that, Descartes showed his firm conviction in the duality of the world.[9]

Mind and Matter as parts of the Mechanical System

After Kant it is Descartes who, for the first time in the domain of the Western philosophy, insisted on the importance of the divisions between man and nature. In his insistence there lied an impropriety. He was unable to offer a reasonable evidence about the dualism of mind and matter. His successors, especially Spinoza and Leibniz fulfilled the gap by constructing theories of ultimate reality. Those theories did not provide much room for the recognition of the qualitative distinction between man and nature. The Jewish philosopher, Spinoza, asserted that the universe, including physical things and mind is, ultimately, a single substance. It may indiscriminately be called either God or Nature. Spinoza definitely holds that the world of mind, like the world of matter, is a part of the whole mechanical system, and not a plurality of free individuals. He thus upheld a conception of the world order in which the whole as well as parts are devoid of individuality, personality and freedom. We regard those qualities exactly as essential to morality and religion. Spinoza couldn't explain how the mental and the physical sides of the universe stand in relation to each other within the single mechanical system conceived by him. While trying to avoid the partition of the unity of the world-order, Spinoza tried to maintain the integrity of the two sides, the matter and mind. He finally asserted that the two sides of the universe were the attributes of the single substance, God.[10]

Let us come back briefly to Descartes again. His distinction between mind regarded as essentially characterized by *thought,* and matter conceived as having extension or space as its essence. He went further. For reasons of his own, he came to hold that the thought and extension were contraries. With the result that the unquestionable anomaly of the relation between man and nature is completely obliterated. It does not matter whether thought and extension are contraries or not to each other. Descartes' understanding of the relation between man and nature seems to be a mistake on account of his views on this relation dualistically.

However, the mistake of Descartes repeats itself in the case of Kant in so far as he comes to construe the dichotomy of man and nature. The dualism of man endowed with freedom and nature, is conceived governed by the principle of mechanical determinism. Of course, Kant admits that man is also a part of nature and as such is as subject to the principle of mechanical determinism as is nature. This amounts to the understanding of human existence itself dualistically and thereby rendering it unintelligible. In consequence, Kant lands himself in a difficulty similar to that of Descartes. He regards freedom as the essence of human existence in one of it other aspects, as well as the essence of the existence of Nature.[11]

So far we have presented the views of some principal Western philosophers. In their opinion the reality consists of some kind of duality, though there exists a unitary factor that binds the duality into one whole—reality. Now we would like to discuss the concept of duality from the point of view of the Eastern philosophers. In the quest of reality and in seeking the path of *Nirvana or Mukti,* they seem to have discussed it more passionately.

Eastern Approach

The *Upanishads*, the ancient Indian literature reported to contain the highest truths, were revealed by the sacred Guru to 5-6 disciples at a time. The Guru explained that the ultimate truth or reality is composed of two—'Brahman' and 'Atman', described as the 'two pillars' on which rests nearly the whole edifice of Indian philosophy. Brahman, as prayer is, what manifests itself in audible speech. 'From this should have been derived later the philosophic significance that it bears in the Upanishads, viz., the primary cause of the universe—what *bursts forth* spontaneously as nature as a whole and not as mere speech only.'[12]

Atman and Brahman

The explanation of these two words is not quite certain. In all probability *atman* originally meant 'breath'. Then it meant as whatever constitutes the essential part of anything, particularly of man, i.e., his self or soul. Thus, each of these terms has its own independent significance: The clear meaning of 'Brahman' is the ultimate source of the outer world, while that of *atman* is the inner self of man. There is something remarkable about these terms. Though they are entirely different in their original connotation, they come to be prevailingly used as synonymous—each significantly alike the eternal source of the universe including nature as well man. That means the outer reality was identified with the inner. By such an identification at last reached the goal of man's long quest after unity—a goal that left all mythology far behind and was truly philosophical.[13]

It is quite important, at this juncture, to deal at some length how this identification was brought about. In finding out the central essence of the individual as distinguished from the physical frame with which it is associated, *atman,* during the course of time, was known as soul or self. Though the method to reach the term 'soul' was subjective, it was arrived at through introspection. In place of the body, breath, etc., that may easily be mistaken for the individual, a deeper principle, that is physical, finally evolved as the essence of man.

From the time of the later *Mantras and Brahmans** people were in the habit of seeking for a correspondence between the individual and the world. They tried to discover for every important feature of the individual, an appropriate counterpart in the other. It represented an effort to express the world in terms of the individual. This notion of parallelism between the individual and the world runs throughout the later Vedic period and is found in the *Upanishads* also. *Atman,* soul or self that is the inmost truth of an individual, became as the cosmic soul, the inmost truth of the world. When the universe came once to be conceived in this manner, its self became the only Self. The other selves were gradually regarded as, in some way, individuals with it.

There was all along another movement of thought almost complementary to the one we have narrated here above. It traced the visible universe to a single source named Brahman. The method used was objective, for it proceeded by analyzing the outer world and not by looking inward as in line of speculation of which *atman* was the central theme. In accordance with the general spirit of Indian thought, several conceptions were evolved—each more satisfying than the previous one, and to describe the universe and Brahman was last in the series of solutions.[14]

At the same stage in the evolution of thought, this primal source of the universe, viz., Brahman got identified with its essence, that is, *atman.* Thus, two independent thought process—one resulting from the desire to understand the true nature of man and the other, that of the objective world—became blended. That blending led at once to the discovery of the unity for that there had been such a prolonged search. The physical world, according to the *atman* doctrine, is only

---

* The *Mantras* and *Brahmans* are among the **Upanishadic** literature.

the not-self. Now it becomes reducible to the self. The blending or fusing of the two such outwardly different but inwardly similar conceptions into one, is the main point of Upnishadic teaching. It is expressed in the 'great sayings' (mahavakya) like 'that thou art', 'I am Brahman' or by the equation Brahman = atman. That means the individual and the world as well, are the manifestation of the same reality and both at the bottom are one.[15]

In order to clarify the concept of Brahman further, more explanations are needed at this point. The chief Vedantic schools may be classified as either absolutistic or theistic. The former representing Brahman, the ultimate reality, as an impersonal principle and the latter as a personal God. These schools of Vedanta are three, known as Advaita, Visistadvaita and Dvaita, predominantly associated with the names of Samkara, Ramanuja and Madhava respectively. We shall confine our attention and discussion mainly to Advaita, thus to Samkara. His approach to Brahman and Atman is in line with our stream of thought, i.e., initially dualism but ultimately unity. It is a pity that the exact period when Samkara lived and worked is not known. He is existed about the close of the 8th and beginning of the 9th century (788–820). In all his works, he subscribes himself as a pupil of Govinda. It is quite unfortunate that Samkara is stated to have died at the age of 32. But he left behind many works, both in verse and prose, and many commentaries on the Vedanta Sutra and almost all the classical Upanisads.[16]

Samkara regards all diversity as being illusion *(mithya)*. But at this point it is very important to grasp correctly the significance of so describing it. Samkara's conception of real *(sat)* is that of eternal being, and Brahman is the sole reality of that type. His conception of the unreal *(asat)* is that of absolute nothing. The world, in all its variety, is neither of the one type nor of the other. It is not real in this sense, for it is anything but eternal. Nor is it unreal in the sense defined, for it clearly appears to us as no non-entity. This is the reason why the world is described in Advaita as other than the real and the unreal or as an illusory appearance. For example, the serpent that appears where there is only a rope is neither existent nor non-existent. It is psychologically given *(prasiddha)*, but cannot be logically established *(siddha)*. In other words, the things of the world though not ultimately real, are yet of a certain order of reality.[17]

While the above description of the physical world in Advaita is a kind of general conception, their description of individual self is very different. But before explaining this difference, it is quite imperative to draw attention of the readers to an important distinction between two types of illusion in common experience. It is well explained with the help of the previously given example. A person sees a 'rope' as a 'serpent' at a distance, while at a closer proximity the rope reveals itself to him as a rope only. The latter knowledge affirms the existence of something which contradicts that something appeared before. He says to himself or feels when he discovers his error; "It is rope, not a serpent." This illusion consists in mistaking a given object for another that is not given. Now such types of illusions illustrate the difference in the manner in which, according to Samkara, one and the same 'Brahman' comes to appear both as the world and as the individual self *(jiva)*. It gives rise to the illusion of the world as the rope does to that of serpent in the above referred example. The ultimate truth, as realized by *Jivanmukta,* denies the world while affirming the underlying reality of Brahman, with which we may be constantly, though not consciously, in touch. The individual self, on the other hand, is not illusory in this sense. It is Brahman itself appearing through media *(upadhi)* like the internal organ that all are elements relating to the physical world, and as such, are illusory. When this fact is realized in one's own experience, what is denied is not the jiva as a spiritual entity. It is only certain aspects of it such as its finitude and its separateness from other selves. We cannot therefore, say that the individual self is false *(mithya),* as we may that the world is false. We can only say that it is not truly the agent, the enjoyer, etc.[18]

Thus, Samkara lays particular emphasis and brings out clearly what is meant by the identity of the *Jiva* and *Brahman* that is of fundamental importance to the doctrine. The 'Jiva' is not false or illusory as the world is, for if it were, there would be none to be saved and the whole teaching of the Upanishads would then be nullified. Salvation implies survival. The liberated 'Jiva' is not lost in Brahman but understands Brahman in all its purity. Thus, the Advaitic world-view is that Brahman is the sole reality—whether it appears as the objective universe or as the individual subject. The objective universe is an illusory manifestation of Brahman, while the latter is Brahman itself appearing under the limitations that form part of that illusory universe.[19]

Four Important Concepts of Advaita

At this point we would like to present four important concepts of the Advaitins to understand their explanations on duality more clearly. Brahman and Jiva have already been discussed to some length above. Still more understanding of these concepts is required to know how the Advaitins comprehend the material and the spiritual extend arguments to stand to their reasoning. These four concepts are: *Maya, Brahman, Sagun-brahman, and Jiva.* Out of the four—one is the concept of nature, as we may term it. The remaining three are the concepts of spirit. Let us examine them separately.

Maya

It has already been stated that the external world is unreal, but it is not therefore to be taken chaotic. Empirically it is a cosmos and Samkara often speaks of it as exhibiting spatial, temporal and casual order. That it is incessantly undergoing change is obvious. However, the change is not total and it involves an element of persistence. These two circumstances suggest that there exists unity in diversity and it also admits to be thought of in two stages, i.e. that the diversity is latent and manifest as well. The Sankhya-Yoga admits that the element of unity is prominent but not that of diversity, as Prakriti. The latter phase, in which that element is obscured by diversity, is what we all understand to be the everyday world. But the physical world does not comprise with the whole universe as there is a spiritual element also in it. So far the explanations given by the Sankhya and the Advaita are similar. But at this point a divergence appears between the two doctrines. It is mainly in regard to the relation between matter and spirit framing the universe as known to us. That divergence is presented here under.

The Sankhya-Yoga, one of the important schools of Indian philosophy, holds that Purusha *(spirit)* and Prakriti *(matter)* are the only reality. They are responsible in constituting the universe as they have close relationship with each other. Thus, Sankhya-Yoga fails to explain satisfactorily the relationship between matter and spirit—more so that they are two identified entities and at the same time capable to constitute the universe. The Advaita definitely denies that there can be any relation at all between two such disparate entities as spirit and matter. However, our investigation of experience leads us to the conclusion that they are not only together but are often identified with each other. For example, when a person says "I am playing", the act of playing is clearly a feature implying the physical body. At the same time it is predicated of the person's self that is spiritual. The only explanation conceivable to it is that their association must be simply appearance or, in other words, the relation between them is ultimately false. Samkara, in his preamble to the commentary on the *Vedanta Sutra,* reflects, "The Self or the I-element is so opposed to the non-self or thou-element that they can never be predicated of each other." An important corollary to this conclusion is that one of the relata is unreal. Both cannot be regarded as unreal, because in that case, all the three elements—the two relata and the relation, becomes false. The Advaitin, therefore, takes for granted that it is matter that ultimately is false. This is the reasoning by which the Advaita arrives at the conclusion that the physical world is only an appearance. There exists the fundamental difference from Sankhya Yoga. This leads us to conclude that the Prakriti is also false, or, in Advait terminology, "other than real and unreal".

In the Advaita doctrine it is known as *Maya*. The term *Prakriti* may be applied to it so long that here it is neither real nor independent of spirit as in Sankhya Yoga. That is to state that if *Maya* explains the world, we would need to seek for its further explanation. The Advaitins take it neither real nor unreal, but it is not ultimate, and that entity that explains it, is spirit... That may also mean that the *evolutes* of *Maya* are more or less the same as those of Prakriti in Sankhya Yoga.

Brahman

We have already briefly discussed Brahman above. Still more explanations are required to clarify the Advaitin's point of view in that respect. We had started that Prakriti is the source of the physical universe. We also arrived at the conclusion that the source, being unreal necessarily implies a ground, viz., Spirit. This Spirit, what

Brahman or the Advaitic Absolute signifies, is the ultimate basis of everything. Whatever reality the world manifests, is derived from it. It has already been stated that in negating the world, we are simply denying its existence apart from or independently of Brahman. To mention the same in a different or alternative phrase it could also be that the world is not a part or phase of Brahman but an appearance of it. That may also mean that the world is an 'actual' change of *Maya* or that it is a change of Brahman as well. This leads us to understand that *Maya* is conceived as really undergoing change in the process of manifesting the world. But Brahman in the same process is conceived as changeless. Thus, we may consider Brahman the cause of the universe also, in the same sense when a rope is the cause of the serpent as given in the example of illusory experience. Just as there wouldn't be any serpent without the rope, there would not be any world or *Maya* without spirit. So, spirit is the only reality and the rest is either *Maya* or its transformation. Although the universe cannot be explained without Brahman, He is devoid of 'unity and diversity' that are the characteristic features of the empirical world. Brahman transcends all empirical attributes as stated and taught in the famous Upanishadic dictum "Not this, not this" *(neti neti)*. Hence it is *nirguna,* or regarded as devoid of qualities. If Brahman is devoid of qualities or attributes, the question arises whether such entity is not sheer abstraction. Samkara, recognizing the importance of this argument, refutes Upanishadic teaching that was in vogue in his time. It was that 'Brahman is universal Being'. Samkara does not view the ultimate reality as objective, but only as identical with the individual self. And this conception also secures the maximum certainty to the reality of Brahman. Nothing can possibly carry greater certainty with it than one's belief in the existence of oneself. "A man may doubt of many things, but he can never doubt of his own being," for that very act of doubting would affirm its own existence. It is thus eventually through something in ourselves that we are able to judge of reality and unreality, says Samkara. But it does not mean that the Self is known to us completely. It also does not remain wholly unknown, being our own self. We also need to remember in this connection 'What it meant by Brahman as featureless?' It is that it transcends the distinction between substance and attribute.[20]

Sagun-brahman

The foregoing discussion leads us to understand that Brahman and *Maya* may each be represented as the cause of the universe, though in different senses. If we look upon them as 'together' constituting the source of the world, their combination becomes to be known as the qualified *(saguna)* Brahman, that comprehends all the diversity of experience. Thus, Brahman may be conceived in two stages—as cause and effect. In the former, the diversity is latent but in the latter it is manifest. When Brahman is mingled with the falsity of Maya, it descends to the phenomenal level. As a result it is designated as the lower *(apara)* Brahman. It then forms the cosmic parallel of the individual self or the ego. Each is Brahman itself with an unreal adjunct; only the adjunct is all-comprehensive in one case, while it is finite in the other. The finite adjunct of the individual self is sometimes designated as *avidya* (ignorance) to construct it with the cosmic Maya of the qualified Brahman. In this way, *Maya* is the whole of which many *avidyas* associated with the individual selves, are parts. Now, these *avidyas* play very important roles in individual lives. Just as the whole universe is the effect of *Maya*, the portions of the universe, that constitute the accompaniments of an individual self, like his physical body and the internal organs, are regarded by the Advaitins as derived from the *avidya* of that particular self. Whatever distinction appears to be there between the ego and the qualified Brahman, is entirely due to the differing adjuncts. The egos are not distinct from one another or from the qualified Brahman. The connotations of *jiva* and the qualified Brahman are quite different. Yet, this kind of identity of denotations of the two—*jiva* and the qualified Brahman, is the Advaitic interpretation of "That thou art" (*Tat tvamsi*). It does not mean, as it is so often represented to do, that man and the qualified Brahman (God), are as such one. According to Advaita, such an attitude, would be considered as blasphemous. So it would be according to any other religion.

The qualified Brahman, when personified, becomes God or *Isvara* of Advaita. Like that, God also may be represented as the cosmic parallel to the finite individual self. The distinction between the individual self and God is entirely one of adjuncts. In that distinction God remains unaffected by any of the evil consequences of association with a finite adjunct, such as shallow love or hate. There is no place for attachment and although God is attached to all that, but is really never attached to anything.[21]

An ancient Sanskrit verse unfolds: 'One should give up attachment; but if that be not possible, one might cultivate it, but it should be equal attachment for all.' There is a popular belief among the people who have faith in Vedanta, that 'God is the creator of the universe. *Maya* is the power *(sakti)* that helps Him in creating the universe.' In this form, God (Brahman) becomes the material as well as the efficient cause of the universe. It has already been stated in this chapter before. He is also sometimes known as the great Magician who brings forth out of himself the entire spectacle of the universe. He has been compared with a magician as he never gets deluded by that spectacle, as others often do. He never fails in realizing his actual character. So the evil does not touch him. The *Gita*, one of the most widely read religious books, throws more light on another popular concept of *Isvara*. It unfolds:

> *Think of the Supreme Person as one who knows everything, who is the oldest, who is the controller, who is smaller than the smallest, who is the maintainer of everything, who is beyond any material conception, who is inconceivable, and who is always a person. He is luminous like the sun, beyond this material nature, transcendental.*[22]

The concept of the Supreme contained in the above verse is widely accepted by the people in the East. He is not impersonal or void, for how one can meditate on something that is impersonal or void. He is the origin of everything and everything is born of Him. He is also the Supreme controller of the universe. What is really important is not that there is a qualified Brahman or God, but He is the Absolute, who is the Ultimate. These Vedantic conceptions are like stepping-stones to the weaker among the disciples and people. They help them in rising to a true conception of the ultimate reality.

Jiva

We have already spoken of the *Jiva* in its relation to Brahman. Therefore, there is not much to add here about it. Still a few things need to be taken care of to clarify its complex character. The *Jiva* or ego, like the qualified Brahman, is also complex in its character as it is a blend of the self and not-self. The latter element is *avidya* (ignorance), that corresponds to *Maya* in the case of the qualified Brahman. Although both the Jiva and God are alike complex in character, there is a vast difference in them. *Maya* is taken to be the power of God and is seen associated with the Brahman. The *Jiva* feels associated with its off-shoots of internal organs *(antah-karana)*, specially when in the state of dream. When it is awake, it feels associated with its physical body due to *avidya*. The two elements in it are wrongly identified with each other, while they are not in the other. It is due to this wrong identification (accepting dualistic conception ignorantly) that all the confusions and troubles of life arise. It is in this complex form that the Self functions as a subject. Consequently the false identity of the Self and the not-self becomes prior to all kinds of experience. The Advaitins consider it a necessary precondition of the Self. Due to its complex nature, that presupposes *avidya* or ignorance, liberation or freedom depends upon the overcoming of *avidya* by transcending the notion of the ego. Thus, though it seems quite paradoxical, if man wants to be himself, he must get beyond himself. Only then a person would get liberated. The (liberated) *jiva* is the jiva that is not related to any of its adjuncts. It would be a true *jiva* and would be viewed in its true character. When it reaches that stage, it would be similar or just like the Advaitic conception of the *Saksin,* or "witness"—aloof from all of them (adjuncts). Without becoming a witness, or being aloof from its false identity, the Self cannot become free or a Jivan-mukta or liberated. The true *jiva* is 'pure consciousness', the "seeing light", and is virtually the same as Brahman, contends the Advaitins. It can be described as the 'transcendental ego', distinguished from the jiva or the empirical ego. The *jiva* conceived as 'pure consciousness' is never limited by its internal organs and confounded with the wrong knowledge or *avidya*.[23]

Thus, *avidya* or ignorance is the sole cause of the Self's miseries and its confinement with the notions of duality. It is, therefore, necessary for the Self to distinguish itself from the empirical ego and transcend to a level of pure consciousness. The *Bhagvad Gita* also contends with similar notions. It indicates that when the Self believes that it is the product of matter, it cannot be liberated. The *Gita* unfolds:

When our consciousness is contaminated by matter, this is called our conditioned state. The false ego is the belief that one is the product of matter. One who is absorbed in this bodily conception, as Arjuna was, must get free from it. This is preliminary for one who wants liberation. Freedom from material consciousness is called mukti. In Srimad-Bhagavatam, also, mukti is used to mean liberation from the material concepts, and a return to pure consciousness. The whole aim of Bhagavad Gita is to teach us to reach this state of pure consciousness.[24]

Empirical World is Impermanent

Our discussions on the concept of dualism would, perhaps, remain incomplete if we do not include here the views of a well-known ancient Indian philosophical school, Buddhism. It recognized the existence of the material world as impermanent. Therefore, Buddha emphasized to transcend it to reach the realm devoid of suffering and frustration. It could be done by overcoming our attachments and desires. For this purpose, he took up the traditional Indian concepts of *Maya, Karma* and *Nirvana* and gave them a fresh dynamic relevant psychological interpretation. We have already discussed the concepts of *maya* (ignorance), *kaya* (material body) and *chitta* (immaterial mind) in our first chapter when defining the meaning of the Self. The concepts of *Karma* and *Nirvana* will be taken care of when we will reflect upon Buddha's procedure to attain freedom or *Nirvana*. When Buddha got enlightenment, perhaps his first reactions towards the objective world would have been strange. He must have thought that our desires, being hooked up with the attractions of the world, lead us to frustration as nothing seemed to him permanent in this world. He, therefore, reached the conclusion that our desires and identification with the mortal objects would always give us only a short lived and impermanent happiness. He always emphasized that all 'things' and the world as well, were impermanent. So he insisted on freedom from the fascination of not only the physical world, but the authority of the spiritual masters too, including his own. He believed that it is up to every individual to tread this way to the end through his or her own efforts. The Buddha's last words on his deathbed are characteristic of his world-view and of his attitude as a teacher. Before he passed away he said: Decay is inherent in all compounded things; strive on with diligence.[25]

Such a conclusion about the world must have flashed on to Buddha by his 'reason' and experience. The fact is that these truths vitally affect our understanding of the common problems of life. One of the truths he conceived was that everything as we know it, is in constant change. The universe of our experience is not a static affair but a dynamic process. Things arise or come in existence through the interaction of the factors necessary to produce them. They maintain themselves carefully for a longer or shorter time, but sooner or later their existence ends. This sort of observation must have led Buddha to conclude that 'decay and dissolution' are inherent in the very nature of finite existence. As a result, the ills bound up with these phases of change, are brought to us along with other forms of existence. So all of us and those whom we love, are subject to illness, old age, sorrows, frustration and death. Thus, no security or happiness is possible that is not really grounded in the acceptance of the principle of change. In the light of such principles and as a result of his day to day experience, Buddha developed a new framework of thought. It led him to the rejection of the two basic concepts—*Brahman* and *atman,* that had been developing in India for such a long time. Not only that, he went one step further. He believed that person had no substantial soul. The popular belief in transmigration, was therefore, also rejected. It was perhaps due to this sort of belief that the Buddhist masters did not like to give any clear answer to the monks' questions, inquiring about the meaning of the Self. The basic truths that Buddha had finally discovered were:

1. Existence is unhappiness.
2. Unhappiness is caused by selfish desires and longings.
3. Selfish cravings can be destroyed.
4. Destruction can be avoided by following Buddha's 'eight-fold path'.

One of the striking things in these findings of Buddha is that there is no reference of anything transcending the human experience. He did not mention any superhuman entity or aid in resolving man's problems. So God does not exist as far as Buddha's analysis of the human problems is concerned. What Buddha is presenting to the world is that surely there are difficult problems (sufferings). Men and women need to confront them and free themselves from any unrealistic hopes and cosmological theories that lie beyond the verification of human experience.[26]

The important thing is that Buddha perhaps never mentioned that the world did not exist. What he said, was that the world is transitory. As change is taking place continually, we are subject to experience suffering on account of decay and destruction. Who is the one experiencing that suffering? It is a question to reassert man's existence and existence of something that is finer in him. Therefore, though Buddha did not accept any theory of soul's existence independently, he could also not explain very convincingly his own theory of a 'continuous flow of consciousness'. How could that flow of consciousness be the experiencer of the objects of the impermanent world? In the first few centuries after the death of Buddha, several Great Councils were held by the leading Buddhist monks. The fourth of these councils took place in Sri Lanka (Ceylon) in the first century. The memorized doctrines, that so far had been passed on orally, were for the first time recorded in writing. This record written in the Pali language, is known as the Pali Canon. It forms the basis of the orthodox Hinayana school. The Mahayana school, another important school of Buddhism besides the Hinayana, is based on a number of so called sutras and scriptures of huge proportions. The first exponent of the Mahayana school and one of the greatest thinkers among the Buddhist preachers, was Ashvaghosha. He lived in the first century AD. He formulated fundamental thoughts of the Mahayana Buddhism and summed them up in a small book named, *The Awakening of Faith.* It is considered as a principal authority on Mahayana Buddhism.[27]

In line with Buddha's findings, the Mahayana school confirms that the physical world is an illusory product of *avidya,* that is the cause of all human suffering and misery. Thus, a constant rejection of the physical world, on the grounds that it is impermanent, is reported in the Buddhist writings. In a way it is also a confirmation that physical world exists, for nothing would be subject to change if it were not there. The Jaina system of thought does not reject the notion of atoms or the reality of the physical world. They do recognize the existence of different categories of jivas. They are known as *tir jivas* that have five sense organs and known with different names. The

Jainas also provide quite elaborate explanations of soul's existence as its various characteristics are subject to human experience. It has already been stated in the first chapter of this book. Therefore, the Jainas belief in dualism cannot be totally denied.

All the above discussions relating to the doctrine of dualism, lead us to conclude that both the Western and the Eastern philosophers accept the existence of the world by their manner of constantly rejecting it, for that which does not exist, need not to be rejected. Some take it to be illusory but perceived by us on account of our 'ignorance'. Others reckon it to be transitory, but perceived as changeless and permanent due to our *avidya.* In this way the reason of our deception and viewing it as real, is mainly caused by our ignorance or *avidya.* Why is it so that the human beings are endowed with 'ignorance'? Is it a prerequisite to man's creation and existence, or is it donned on him without his desire, are some of the questions worth analyzing. But before we proceed to know the cause of *avidya* that probably stops us from knowing ourselves thoroughly, let us briefly retrospect the views of the Eastern and the Western thinkers on dualism contained in this chapter.

Retrospection

From the Western point of view the reality consists of as 'Ideas'. The 'being' of things is a subordinate and a defective being. It is founded on the 'being' of the Ideas in which the things share. Plato believes that a true being lives in the Ideas, that are not directly accessible to one's consciousness. They are precisely not in the world.

Nevertheless one knows them in some way. They are within him, as persons have seen, to know the things. Thus, Plato does not seem to be much clear about his own hypothesis of the doctrine of dualism. It (confusion) appears from the expression, 'nevertheless one knows them in some way'. What that some way could be, is not clear to us. Let us also examine Socrates' position in this respect. Through the myth he reveals that the soul, in its original state, can be compared with a chariot drawn by the two horses. He narrates that the troubles arise in guiding the flight of the two horses, and the soul falls. The horses lose their wings and the soul becomes incarnated in a body. Well, it is just a myth. It cannot lead us to know 'how after the wings are lost, the soul becomes incarnated.' It appears to be merely a conjecture. It cannot be accepted rationally. Spinoza asserts that the entire universe, including physical things and mind, is ultimately a single substance that he indiscriminately calls God or nature. He holds that both, the world of mind and world of matter, are parts of the whole mechanical system and not a plurality of free individuals. He is not able to explain how the mental and the physical sides of the universe stand in relation to each other within the single mechanical system. His predecessor Descartes, who insists on the importance of the divisions between man and nature, is unable to offer a reasonable evidence about the dualism of matter and mind. Kant is also unable to offer us a satisfactory account of the dichotomy of man and Nature. According to Kant, man is endowed with freedom and is also part of nature, conceived to be governed by the principle of mechanical determinism. That means he is also subject to the principle of mechanical determinism.

The Advaitins visualize duality in term of various concepts, such as Brahman, qualified Brahman, *Maya* and *Jiva*. Samkara speaks of external or empirical world as real and unreal. At many occasions he speaks of it as exhibiting spatial, temporal and casual order. Therefore, it is obvious that unceasingly it is undergoing change. The change is not total and involves a persistent element. All this suggests that there lays unity in the diversity. The Advaitins also hold that the physical world does not exhaust the universe and there is a spiritual element also in it that is the Self or *atman*. At this point, a divergence appears between the Advaitins and the Sankhya Yoga, which is in regard to the relation between spirit and matter as the constituents of the universe. The Sankhya Yoga recognizes that the *Purusha* and *Prakrit* are two different entities but are instrumental in creating this universe. The Advaitins refute this approach. They consider that 'the Self or the I-element is so opposed to the not-self that they can never be predicated of each other.'

The Buddhists reckon the empirical world as impermanent and, therefore, if someone conceives it as real, it would be due to one's *avidya* or ignorance. In place of the soul, the Buddhists reckon that there is only a 'stream of consciousness'. After death, it continues in another body just as a burning flame lights up another flame in the same lamp.

The Jainas accept that the existence of the physical world is temporary. They contend that there are many kinds of *jivas* that possess different sense organs. The Jainas also hold that avidya plays an important role in confusing man to know the true nature of reality. Consequently, it brings him suffering. The above discussions lead us to conclude the following points from the philosophers' thoughts presented so far:

1. Most of the Western philosophers believe that spiritual as well as the physical worlds exist. *The spiritual transcends the physical* in the sense that the material world is known or recognized by the mind or spirit. So it is more real. Both, Democritus and Plato acknowledge the reality of perception. They also accept that 'thought' is the real source of knowledge. Parmenides and the philosophers of his time believe that the true being does not reside in things. It resides outside of them in the Ideas as the being of things is defective or is subordinate to the being of Ideas.

Similarly, Plato and Aristotle believe that the world of spirit is more real. Aristotle considers it a living force that brings realization to the human body. Kant holds that the world of appearance is characterizable by *knowability par excellence,* and the world of reality is *unknown and unknowable.* Rene Descartes holds that nature is fundamentally divided into two separate and independent realms—mind and matter. His famous sentence, *Cogito ergo sum,* "I think so I exist," leads him and the other Western thinkers to equate their identity with their mind instead of with the whole organism. According to Descartes reality has two fundamental divisions—matter and mind, but mind is in complete control of the whole organism. Thus, the reality is more akin to the spirit rather than the matter. Invariably 'reason' is the best instrument to reach that conclusion.

2. In the process of rejecting the external world, the Vedantics and the Buddhists recognize it indirectly. The Jainas accept it almost directly. The *Bhagwad Gita* accepts and rejects it in the manner of the Vedantics. Thus, the Eastern philosophers, under the Vedantic spell, *visualize the reality as Pure Spirit,* which in other words is the Brahman itself.

As the thought process developed, ideas started getting maturer. With that the primal source of the universe, viz., Brahman, was identified with its inmost essence, that is *atman.* The other concepts of the Vedantics may initially look different, but they belong to only one reality, i.e. Brahman. Thus, the Advaitins definitely denies that there can be any relation at all between two such disparate entities as spirit and matter. They visualize, mainly through the mystic procedures, that reality precipitating into four concepts, submerges into one. Peter Fingesten, explaining the Vedanta concept of reality states:

> *The Vedantic School is purely monistic. It does not teach the existence of the individual soul as distinct from the universal soul. It formulated the doctrine of maya, or illusion; the universe exists, but it is only the illusion of the one eternal essence which is at once existence, knowledge, and joy.*[28]

Both the Eastern and the Western philosophers agree that *illusion, avidya or maya is the chief cause of man's misunderstanding the nature of reality.* Plato, narrating the Socratic myth says, 'if the soul has seen the Ideas, even though only briefly, this body will be human and not bestial'. The soul is simply not able to see Ideas on account of its ignorance. It is also the reason of the soul's falling from the heaven. In the 'Simile of the Cave' the chained-man is equated to the 'ignorant-man' who is unable to see rightly and when he is free from the chains, he sees the real world outside. Socrates always equated ignorance with the evil. He thought that if a man stole from his neighbour and turned himself into a thief and a liar, it was because he expected to get good out of it. No one went after evil knowingly. Therefore, he believed that 'what a terrible thing it was to be ignorant—to be fooled about what was good. No matter how well-made your body, how brilliant your mind, if you were ignorant of Good, your whole life would go in the wrong direction."[29]

The Vedantics repeatedly emphasize that *avidya* causes illusion and thus leads the Self to identify itself with the body or material world. 'The finite adjunct of the individual self is sometimes designated as *avidya* to contrast it with the cosmic *Maya* of the qualified Brahman. In this view, Maya is the whole of which the many *avidya,* associated with the individual selves, are parts or phases. The *Bhagwad Gita* contends that 'at every moment, the texture and quality of our thoughts are directly conditioned and controlled by our desires. Thoughts expressed in the outer world-of-objects, become man's actions. Thus, in this chain-of-'ignorance', constituted of desires, thoughts and actions, each one of us is caught and bound.[30]

Chinmayananda, elaborating the term *avidya* states:

> *If we observe them (desires, thoughts and actions) a little more closely, we find that these are not so many different factors, but are, in fact, different expressions of one and same spiritual ignorance. This ignorance (avidya), when it functions in the intellect, expresses itself as desires. When the desires, which are nothing other than the 'ignorance, ' function in the mental zone, they express themselves as thought.*[31]

The Buddha did not recognize the Self as an independent entity. It is clear from the discussions of the masters and the monks. Some of their discourses have been quoted in the first chapter under the section 'The Eastern Approach'. One of the basic truths he discovered is that there is suffering in the world. Suffering is caused on account of our ignorance. Ignorance makes us believe that the world is real though it is changing every moment. Therefore, *avidya* plays a very important role in man's life for it causes illusion and consequently brings misery and suffering.

The Jainas are of the opinion that the soul, though it passes through various stages of birth and death, must not be understood in the shape of habits and attitudes. It is as an independent entity, which is spiritual, immaterial, permanent and eternal in the midst of all changes. If it is taken to be the part of the physical body possessing habits and attitudes, it is on account of our ignorance or *avidya*.

The Western and Eastern philosophers seem to dilute the issue of duality in favour of the Self. All of them have a firm conviction that there is always something, which is instrumental in blurring man's vision of his own self. It then leads him into confusion, and consequently makes him plunge into a world of suffering and misery.

The questions, 'why does man suffer and act erroneously' and 'why does he not know himself properly,' are some of the important issues related to his limited knowledge about himself. If ignorance is the main cause of our suffering, can we dispel it from our lives easily? Let us, therefore, discover the ways proposed by the leading philosophers of the world in that respect. Let us find out whether there are some answers to the above questions so that our present and future may become more wholesome and ignorance and suffering may go away from our lives. Is there really any process or path that could lead us to peace and ever lasting happiness? All this will form the content of our next chapters.

References

The Concept of Dualism

1. Fritjof Capra, *The Tao of Physics,* p. 7.
2. W. Windelband, *A History of Philosophy,* pp. 104–105.
3. Windelband, *A History of Philosophy,* pp. 123–124.
4. Windelband, *A History of Philosophy,* p. 124.
5. Julian Marias, *History of Philosophy,* pp. 46–47.
6. Julian Marias, *History of Philosophy,* p. 47.
7. Julian Marias, *History of Philosophy,* pp. 48–50.
8. Will Durant, *The Story of Philosophy,* p. 69.
9. Capra, *The Tao of Physics,* pp. 8–9.
10. Nikunja Vehari Banerjee, *Philosophy of Reconstruction,* pp. 33–34.
11. Nikunja V. Banerjee, *Philosophy of Reconstruction,* pp.70–79.
12. M. Hiriyanna, *Outlines of Indian Philosophy,* p. 12.
13. Hiriyanna, *Outlines of Indian Philosophy,* pp. 54–55.
14. Hiriyanna, *Outlines of Indian Philosophy,* pp. 55–56.
15. Hiriyanna, *Outlines of Indian Philosophy,* pp. 56–57.
16 R.N. Sharma, *India Philosophy,* pp. 32–38.
17. M. Hiriyanna, *The Essentials of Indian Philosophy,* pp. 155–156.
18. Hiriyanna, *The Essentials of Indian Philosophy,* pp. 156–157.
19. Hiriyanna, *The Essentials of Indian Philosophy,* pp. 158–159.
20. Hiriyanna, *The Essentials of Indian Philosophy,* p. 162.
21. Hiriyanna, *The essentials of Indian Philosophy,* pp. 162–164.
22. Swami Prabhupada, *Bhagavad Gita As It Is,* p. 114.
23. Hiriyanna, *The Essentials of Indian Philosophy,* pp. 165–166.
24. Prabhupada, *Bhagavad Gita As It Is,* p. Intro, xxiv.
25. Fritjo Capra, *The Tao of Physics,* p. 85.
26. Edwin A. Burtt, *Man Seeks the Divine,* pp. 223–225.
27. Fritjo Capra, *The Tao of Physics,* p. 87.
28. Peter Fingesten, *East Is East,* pp. 33.
29. Cora Mason, *The Man Who Dared to Ask,* p. 70.
30. Swami Chinmayananda, *Bhagavad Gita, The Karma Yoga,* p. 12.
31. Chinmayananda, *The Karma Yoga,* p. 12.

3

Concept of Unity

Brihad-aranyaka Upanishad says, "Where there is duality, as it were, there one sees another; there one smells another; there one tastes another....But where everything has become just one's own self, then whereby and whom would one see? Then whereby and whom would one smell? Then whereby and whom would one taste?[1]

This is the final apprehension of the unity of all things. This is what the mystics tell us. The unity is the state of consciousness where one's individuality is dissolved into an undifferentiated oneness and where the world of the senses and the notion of things are transcended and everything is left behind. This is salvation—liberation too. If one is able to attain that state of mind in this life, one would become *jivan-mukta.*

S. Radhakrishnan holds that the state of freedom of mind is the state of unity of the Self. When the Self unites with itself, it gets fully liberated. Liberation does not mean escaping from the world of space and time. Writing the introduction of *The Sacred Writings of the Sikhs,* Radhakrishnan stated: "The aim of liberation is...to be enlightened, wherever we may be. It is to live in this world knowing that it is divinely informed....For those who are no longer bound to the wheel of *samsara,* life on earth is centred in the bliss of eternity. Their life is joy and where joy is, there is creation. They have no country here below except the world itself." Radhakrishnan is indicating to the wheel of *samsara* as a binding factor to person, depriving him from his freedom.[2]

This 'wheel of *samsara*' is constantly moving and thus involving him with the things of the world. This involvement deprives him from knowing that the purpose of life is not indulgence. It is seeking divinity and unity. Is it not on account of man's *avidya* that he is not able to conceive the right meaning of his life? Jiddu Krishnamurti has a better explanation of the wheel of *samsara*. He contends that the spokes of that wheel are also some of the greatest stumbling blocks in our life. In other words they are 'our constant struggles' to reach, to achieve, and to acquire. We are trained from childhood to acquire and to achieve. As a result, the brain cells constantly create and demand this pattern of achievement in order to have physical security. Thus, our minds resolve in endless self-centred thinking, around 'me' and 'my' gains and losses, 'my' desires and despairs, 'my' past and future. This very thinking around 'myself' endlessly self-centred, brings vastly more unhappiness to us all.[3]

We have been talking of man's misery and delusion in our second chapter of this book. We have also indicated that *avidya* (ignorance) and man's attachment to the 'things' of the world have a great spell on him. The truth is that it is so difficult to reject this beautiful world. Even though it may be transient, it looks real and fascinating. We cannot easily mount the intellectual heights Gautama Buddha had attained during his life-time. We cannot also grow suddenly to be so kind and loving as the Christ was. Perhaps we do not have even that much time as Socrates had to analyze the problems. Nor we possess the Socratic courage to ask people the meaning of difficult questions relating to our lives. How can we remove our ignorance when we do not know that we are really ignorant? Even if some of us know it, do we really try to dispel it? Can we easily understand 'the working of our minds' when we are surrounded by pressures created by the newly discovered economic, scientific, educational, social, cultural and moral orders? Do we have eagerness to know ourselves adequately? Do we possess any desire to spare some time for us to stop for a moment from our daily rushing routine to look into ourselves? Will it be possible to acquire any peace of mind, or happiness when we do not have any longing for it? Perhaps it is difficult as all around us a drastic revolution seems to be going on. In spite of it, Edwin A. Burtt, an American educationist, seems to possess some hopes amid all that confusion lurking around us. He remarks:

It is a drastic revolution, and it is world-wide. Perhaps we are as yet only in its early stages. And, among other things, it is a revolution in religion. New faiths are appearing on every hand; old faiths, in their efforts to maintain themselves in the modern world, are undergoing radical reconstruction. It was in such a time of turmoil and anxiety and suffering and hope that all the great historic religions of the world were born, stirring their followers to a new faith and a new energy, a new confidence in themselves and in the divine source of goodness and truth.[4]

Burtt is suggesting us to keep hope in some kind of divine power or something of similar nature that would surely deliver us from our agonies and sufferings. Before a savior is born, I would like to reexamine some of the procedures (which may help bringing unity in us) proposed by the ancient masters. Their outstanding virtuous lives, implicit with humility, intellectual honesty, devotion, love and loyalty, are unparalleled. They stand aloof with others. The posterity can never forget their moral beliefs they practised in their lives.

There could be two possible ways for an individual to meet the challenging situations. One is to accept all the frustration and failure and succumb to fear and hate and react with destructive feelings. The other would be to accept the challenges of life with hope, trust, courage and rejoicing, and to realize a greater good for himself and all humanity. In this respect the role of our ancient religious and moral teachers can never be forgotten. They have always shown us ways to live morally and courageously. They have repeatedly told us to remember that 'this life which is given to us even by accident, is worth living, for it consists of a soul that has divine attributes'. Christ, Buddha, Socrates, Confucius, Rama and Krishna as the ancients, and Jiddu Krishnamurti as the most modern, are some of the best examples in that respect. I shall, therefore, present their principal ideas that have always been considered instrumental in embalming our troubled souls and helping us to seek unity with ourselves.

Greek Master Thinker

Although Socrates left no written records concerning himself, it is quite possible to reconstruct a good account of his virtuous life. The writings of the Greek contemporaries and some research scholars have revived his mighty stature. Both, Aristophanes and Plato caricatured him in their works. They often expressed high praise for him, with special reference to his moral genius, quality of life he lived, and the content of his teachings. Socrates believed that the most important topic that should occupy man's mind was the meaning of good life.

The physicians and the natural scientists of his day were simply struggling to obtain information about the things as they were. Socrates contended that to understand the meaning of human life was a matter of far more significance. Man must know the way that he ought to live. The physical sciences do not tell us about the purpose for which the things exist in the world. They also don't tell us anything about the nature of goodness. They don't reveal what is good or bad and what is morally right or wrong. Therefore, Socrates thought that far more important inquiry would be to do with the knowledge of what makes the good life.

Socrates rejected the popular notions about the Greek gods and their relationship with human beings. He strongly believed that a divine providence had to do with the creation of the world. The purpose towards which it was directed was attainment of a good life on the part of human beings. *Man was not merely a physical being but he also possessed a soul* implicit with divine characteristics.

Socrates' moral philosophy can be briefly expressed in his statement *"virtue is life"*. Whatever years he got to live, he taught that 'a person acquires virtues through the fulfillment of purpose for which he exists.' Therefore, he believed that 'individual is always required to live a virtuous life that he ought to remember and act as well.' This is what he meant by 'the meaning to know thyself.' He further elaborated the precept, 'the meaning to know thyself.' He said that in case of a person, this would mean a harmonious development of the divine elements found in his nature. It would apply to his life as a whole rather than just the present moment or the future that follows. Therefore, each person should remember that the mission of life is not to possess the knowledge of the facts concerning the material universe. It involves an understanding of the soul in relation to the good life only.

Socrates believed that ignorance concerning the good life was the main cause of evil acts of a person. He had a conviction that no one would knowingly do that which was harmful to himself. Only virtue is capable of providing satisfaction to the soul. People do strive to achieve that goal. All do not succeed to reach it because they are ignorant of the fact that all roads do not lead to lasting happiness. Consequently, they tend to pursue sensuous pleasures, public positions, wealth and other goals. They believe that pursuing those goals would bring them the greatest happiness. When they reach any of those goals, they discover that those goals haven't given them real happiness or peace of mind. Therefore, 'every one must understand thoroughly,' Socrates contended, 'that it is through the proper development of one's mind in its pursuit of truth, beauty, and goodness that the goal and purpose of human life can be achieved finally.'[5]

With this clear understanding Socrates became the pioneer philosopher of his time. He believed that the truth can only be revealed if a person knows himself well. This belief was an outcome of Socrates' virtuous life that he lived and experienced by keeping the company of the wise people.

Ever since he was a child he had what he called "the divine sign". Every now and then a feeling came to him. It stopped him from doing whatever he was going to do because it was not good for him to do. What this word 'good' meant, Socrates felt it within, but at first he could not explain it. Gradually he thought that it must have had something to do with happiness. As he grew, he discovered that when he acted as the "sign" told him to, everything turned out good. Soon he came to know that he could depend on the "sign" and obey it even when he did not understand why.[6]

Socrates did not talk much about that "sign". Even later on when he was a grown man, he did not talk about it. It was not a little private god inside him. It was neither a conscience to tell him what was false or true, kind or cruel. It was something beyond that. The sign stopped him from doing even ordinary things, like talking to certain people or visiting certain places. The way Socrates used the sign made a great difference. He took the sign as a simple example of what he must have felt in his heart already. He thought, 'it meant the gods were inspiring him to some good direction, that he must follow.' That also meant, he concluded, 'that the old stories of lying, stealing and angry gods were made up by ignorant persons. Goodness was the mark of the gods and if someone did not agree with it, it was simply his/her imagination.' Keeping it in mind, Socrates acted every time in his life. A best example of it can be quoted when his friend, Crito, comes to him in the jail to advise him to escape.

Crito contends that the case against Socrates is fabricated and therefore, it is right for him to escape from the jail. When Crito is quiet and his excitement subsides, Socrates suggests him to examine the right and wrong of the question. After a while Socrates reminds him of the principles that always laid down the foundations of their decisions. First he picks up Crito's point about what people would say if he escapes. Socrates reflects that one could not judge right and wrong by mere public opinion. If one would listen to the people, one is likely to spoil one's soul just as an athlete would spoil his body if he listens to everyone but his trainer. Then he reminds Crito that simply being alive is not the important thing, but living rightly is important. Socrates does not also believe in returning evil for evil, for evil cannot come from good people. Therefore, he decides to stay in the jail and obeys the city laws that he accepted since birth. He finally tells Crito:

> *This is the voice that is sounding in my ears, Crito, my friend, and the sound of these words is a music that shouts out everything else. If you speak against it—from the way I feel now—you will speak in vain. But still, if you think it will do any good, speak.*[7]

Listening to it Crito says that he has nothing to say any more as whatever Socrates has said is the truth. At that occasion Crito is reminded of an incidence that took place some time back. Both Crito and Socrates after disagreeing at a point of decision, hold back and keep quiet for sometime. Talking any more on it would hurt each other. After a while Socrates resumes the talk and says:

> *Agree with me if I seem to you to say what is true, but if not, pull against everything you have. See to it that I don't deceive you along with myself in my eagerness, and go off like a bee, leaving my sting in you.*[8]

Thus, Socrates went on obeying the "sign" that always told him to do right. In reply to the charges against him, he made a noble defence but it was in line with the manner of life he lived. He presented sufficient evidence to show that the accusations brought against him were without proper foundations. He believed too that the accusers were wrong, yet he never thought to escape from the jail. It was not right to do so. Socrates lived truly and died honestly and courageously. Had he desired, he could have escaped from the jail. He could also get pardon from the court, but he followed the true path only. He acted upon it until he died, for he knew that it was the only meaning of life.

Next to him there is another distinguished philosopher who scaled morally almost the same height what Socrates had reached. He lived a life implicit with 'right' as he thought that it was the only purpose of life. He was Confucius.

Confucius' Golden Rule

Buddhism reached China around the first century AD. Philosophical thought had already culminated to a great height in China by then. The period, which roughly runs from centuries 500-221 BC, is known as the golden age of Chinese philosophy. From the beginning, this philosophy had two complementary systems. As the Chinese are practical people, they possess a highly developed social consciousness. Their philosophical schools were mainly concerned with life in society, moral values, human relations and government as well. Complementary to this, there is another aspect of their philosophy that corresponds to the mystical side of their character. It demands that the highest aim of philosophy should be to guide individual to reach higher plane of consciousness. This is the plane of the sage or the enlightened person who had attained mystical union with the universe.

The sixth century BC witnesses the two sides of the Chinese philosophy. It developed into two distinct philosophical systems, known as Confucianism and Taoism. These two sides of thought represent opposite poles in Chinese philosophy. In China they were always considered two sides of the same coin, and thus complementary to each other. Confucianism derives its name from Kung Fu Tzu, or Confucius (551-479 BC). He was a highly influential teacher of great repute. Confucius had a large number of students, to whom his main function was to transmit the ancient cultural heritage. In doing so he often went ahead. He transmitted the traditional ideals according to his own beliefs and moral concepts.[9]

There was something unique in his personality that appealed to his disciples and followers. As a result, the subsequent generations of Chinese could look back to him 'as the most revered teacher of their past.' It is reported that he was very meticulous in matters of dress, food and social habits. He was a great historical scholar. He believed that both constructive moral insight and sound political system must be based on a wise understanding of the lessons of history. These characteristics were combined with others too. He was full of jollity and humour and would not condemn a joke that was made on him. He loved music and played on the *ch 'in,* a popular Chinese stringed instrument. He disliked insincerity and hypocrisy. He did not boast of his own attainments, and always maintained a dignified self-respect.

During the middle period of his wanderings, around 489 BC, certain basic features of his character and philosophic thought became more popular. It was soon after this that a revealing event occurred. One day Confucius and his followers were surrounded by some soldiers who held them in close custody. The historians report that Confucius and the party gradually got short of food and several members also fell sick. At that occasion Confucius' disciples began to behave in ways that expressed their fear and anxiety. Confucius remained calm and continued to study and to sing on his instrument. Observing Confucius' unusual behaviour, one of his disciples, Tselu, asked him, "Does a superior man sometimes realize when he is in dangerous circumstances?" Confucius replied calmly, "Yes, a superior man is sometimes aware that he is in dangerous circumstances. But when a common man finds himself in danger he forgets himself, and does all sorts of foolish things. "After listening to this remark, the disciple became silent, but other followers were very much impressed. To them Confucius remarked that 'besides studying history, he also contemplates on the basic principle of the Golden Rule.'

Now what was that Golden Rule to which he referred to? The Rule contained:

Do not do to others what you do not wish them to do to you.

What Confucius wanted to tell them, was his own findings about the nature of the truth he discovered during his study and meditation. He discovered that,

> *"...truths by which a man can live whatever the circumstances into which he may fall, truths expressive of his deepest insight and his full moral integrity, truths in following which he knows himself to be in tune with the way of Heaven—truths therefore, in commitment to which a man can overcome all anxiety and fear.*[10]

It seemed to Confucius that the disciples could not completely apprehend what he had said. So he decided to share with them, one by one, the meaning of the Golden Rule. He called Tselu first to converse and share its meaning. Tselu replied that he and his fellow beings were not as wise as to understand its meaning. Then Confucius inquired whether his teachings were wrong! Listening to it another disciple remarked:

"The master's teachings are too great for the people, and that is why the world cannot accept them. Why don't you come down a little from your heights?"

Listening to the disciple's remark Confucius replied:

> *Ah Sze, a good farmer plants the fields but cannot guarantee the harvest, and a good artisan does a skilful job, but he cannot guarantee to please his customers. Now you are not interested in cultivating yourselves, but are only interested in being accepted by the people. I am afraid you are not setting the highest standard for yourself.*[11]

Thus, Confucius always aimed at the highest standards of life. During his time the basic concern was no longer the struggle for life, as it had been in the primitive times. It was instead, the quest for the good life as well as for the finest moral and spiritual realization. Confucius believed that every person was capable to reach the finest moral standards under any sorts of complex conditions. He started stressing the importance of leading a moral life when the political and social situations were at their lowest ebb. His historical knowledge led him to believe that at an earlier time human life was much happier and justice more fully realized. The social and political disorder that prevailed at that time, was rooted in the individual, he thought. Those who were considered 'gentlemen' did not show moral leadership. Far from that they were busy with luxury and base deeds, unsuitable for the 'gentlemen'. Consequently, the common people were immersed into greater subjection, poverty and despair. Was there any solution for such dismal social and personal problems and increasing confusion?

Confucius strongly felt that if there could be any solution to all that deepening social disorder, it must be fundamentally a moral solution. Thus, Confucianism is a constructive ethical philosophy. Confucius, as a master-architect, expects that a real 'gentleman' is the person 'who is endowed with moral insight'. 'He is ready to assume the responsibilities of moral leadership without waiting for others to fill such a role first.' Thus a gentleman is a superior person who initiates the moral growth of the society. He accepts the task of self-renewal, through moral understanding and moral commitment. The person who steadily pursues this course of life will naturally be responsive to the divine harmony.

In Confucianism one of the basic emphases is reverence for the best that has come down to persons from the past. That means, certain modes of conduct that have gradually been established through tradition and custom. These modes help smoothing the social relations, involving expressions of pious emotions that must be preserved and practised sincerely. It would also mean to discipline the rebellious impulses that often lead us to neglect those moral traditions. Such practices would always lead men to realize the unity of spirit that is the highest goal of mankind. In connection with the ideology expressed here above, there is a popular saying which is attributed to Confucius. It says:

In other words it would mean that a man could not express man-to-manness without showing courteous behaviour to others and

> *True manhood consists in realizing your true self and restoring the moral order. If a man can just for one day realize his true self, and restore complete moral order, the world will follow him.*[12]

without respecting genuinely the established traditional manners. In all that expressive behaviour, a sense of flexibility is also implicit. Confucius did not want man to follow the rule blindly. He expected one to be intelligently adjustable to the needs of each new human situation and not to be bound rigidly by any traditional routine. Thus, Confucius expected every gentleman to express moral discrimination in order to realize an ideal 'manness'. That means 'knowing wisely when to be strict and when to show compassion.' It also means 'when to be trustful and when to be cautious, when to assert firmness and when to agree with the wishes of the others.' In short, he must realize the Golden Mean of true courage as compared with the different pairs of extremes. For example, extremes like sentimental pity and callousness, foolhardiness and cowardice, etc., into which a person who lacks the right virtue is likely to fall in.

To follow this kind of wise adaptability to reach right manhood would imply that certain basic principle is followed by a person. This principle must also guide him in all his decisions and acts. It must be a principle that cannot be expressed easily in a few words. Still it helps the superior person (gentleman) to create a moral order by its constant practice. It brings persistent harmony in others too when they practise it. Confucius taught such a principle, that is symbolized by a term *shu,* which usually means "reciprocity". Most of the Western people are familiar with it as the Golden Rule, that can also be expressed in negative form:

Do not do unto others what you do not want others to do unto you.

This kind of universalization of moral conduct has not been very popular in the West as it is quite opposite to the positive form taught in the gospels by Jesus. Jesus said:

Whatsoever you would that men should do unto you, do you even so to them.

Confucius was quite aware of the positive side of his Golden Rule, that can be clarified from quoting some passages from his literature. Confucius, modestly recognizing his own inadequacies, is reported to have stated:

There are four things in the moral life of a man, not one of which have I been able to carry out in my life. To serve my father as I would expect my son to serve me: that I have not been able to do. To serve my sovereign as I would expect a minister under me to serve me: that I have not been able to do. To act towards my elder brother as I should expect my younger brother to act towards me: that I have not been able to do. To be the first to behave towards friends as I would expect them to behave towards me: that I have not been able to do.[13]

The above quotation clarifies Confucius' interpretation of the rule of "reciprocity". It also provides guidance to the person who desires to become a gentleman and embodiment of true manhood. Confucius' ideology contained in the above quotation is important in two respects. One, that it shows the central point in his mind about the role of *shu,* that as he would like others to behave towards him, he will first behave in that manner. He will keep his self-respect and equality maintained. The moral person will not yield to any demands of others so as to act in an inferior manner. Neither he would get exploited. The second aspect is in accord with the ideal man's relationship with the society. In view of these relationships, every normal person can appreciate 'how a just sovereign ought to treat his subject, how an intelligent father ought to treat his son, how a considerate brother ought to treat his younger brother, and how a true friend is expected to treat another friend.' The truth is that in most of these cases every person clearly knows from his own experience how he should behave with others. *Every father knows the feelings of his son as he has been a son first. Similarly, every friend has someone as a friend and knows how he would like to be treated by the other. Every ruler has been subject to authority when he was young.* Thus, Confucius, highlighting the rule of 'reciprocity', amplifies the stature of an 'ideal person' who is really a gentleman. He acts throughout, keeping in mind the Golden Rule. It would, thought Confucius, keep the individual and in turn the family morally stable.

When we summarize Confucius' search for a moral person in view of his Golden Rule, we come to certain conclusion. It is that the gentleman that Confucius had in mind was not anyone else than the virtuous person of Socrates. Yet, perhaps, there is some difference in them. Socrates' vision of a virtuous person is an epitome of moral virtues that were considered invaluable in Socratic Athens. Confucius' gentleman dwells in the ancient China where love for a moral life was a pragmatic reality.

Let us summarize Confucius' views on an integrated moral individual, who is responsible for the stability of a moral family. In turn he is also responsible for creating a stable society:

The truly superior person, according to Confucius, is he (shu) whose virtues are perfected by following the principles contained in the Golden Rule. He will have all the virtues that are responsible to lead him a happy family life every day. He will be sincere in heart and devoted to the right. He will never fail in moral courage, will act responsibly and will be worthy of trust. He will be friendly towards all and will prize wisdom and understanding by developing his insight with the knowledge of the past. He will be open-minded to new situations. He will remain serene and cheerful in mind as he has accepted the universe without desiring more than what he has got, and under all circumstances he will stride to realize moral integrity, which is the highest goal of life. As he is very clear that goodness has its own reward, he will be content with all the vicissitudes and pains that life would offer him."[14]

Thus, Confucius provides a vision of a highly intellectual and moral life that becomes a reality with faith and practice. This is how he aimed for the moral growth of the individual who in turn was responsible for the growth of an integrated moral family and society as well. At this point a question comes to my mind, 'Why was Confucius stressing that a person should lead a moral life and be a gentleman in the right sense?' It was because he himself was a moral human being. Like Socrates he knew perfectly well that the goal of this life could not be other than leading a virtuous life. He did not say much about the divine nature of the soul. Yet he had a transcended vision about the practices that would lead man to the road of the virtuous life. Therefore, he prescribed rules to be practised by the individual to attain all the needed moral values that would make himself and his family happy. It was the true meaning of life which Confucius conceived of.

An Epitome of Morality

In our search towards understanding the meaning to know thyself, I would like to transport the reader from China to India. A few hundred years before Christ, a legendary figure, known as *Rama,* was born to a famous warrior monarch, ***Dashratha.*** He was the ruler of Ayodhya, a great kingdom in the ancient northern India. Ayodhya is situated now in the northern part of Uttar Pradesh (state) in India. Legends reveal that once Dashratha, while fighting with the demons, damaged his chariot in the battle. His third wife, Kaikaye, supported him personally in handling the damaged chariot at that occasion. Besides, she supported him emotionally and morally too. The monarch finally won the battle. Pleased by the queen's demeanour he granted her two boons that she could seek any time she pleased. As the story goes, the queen requested the monarch to grant her the boons right at the time when the old king was about to hand over his kingdom to Rama. One of the boons she asked, was to offer the throne to her own son, Bharat. The other was, that Rama, the son from the monarch's first wife, should be exiled from Ayodhya to the jungles for fourteen years. Rama was not only the eldest son of Dashratha, but was also the rightful owner of the throne after the father. The monarch also loved him very dearly. Since Rama knew that the boons granted by his father, must be fulfilled, he willfuly accepted the vicissitudes in life. In obedience to his father's words given to Kaikyee, he left the kingdom, accompanying with his spouse, Sita, and one of the younger brothers, Laxman. Both Sita and Laxman proceeded to the forests with Rama with their own will as they loved him more than their own lives.

Since our intention is to seek a clear meaning to the precept, *'to know thyself,'* I would like to dwell upon the *ethical aspects of Rama's life.* I shall narrate his story relating to his moral convictions that he never relinquished even though he stayed bare-footed and with meagre clothes in the jungles for fourteen years. In all religions and ethical codes of any society, obedience is considered one of the important virtues. Rama cultivated and practised obedience in all the possible ways even though he faced terrible hardships. Rama's life, therefore, is a story of obedience, fortitude, courage, balance of mind, simplicity and devotion to the traditional values and culture of his time. If he had desired, he could have refused to proceed to the jungles. He could easily take over the throne of his old father by force. It is quite customary in the countries of the other worlds in the past. But he did not do so. His younger brother Bharat, was at his maternal uncle's home at the time Rama had to leave the palace. He did not agree to his mother's wishes. He approached Rama to take him back home. But Rama politely refused to go back as it would mean disobedience to their father and mother Kaikaye as well. He proceeded to the forests, requesting Bharat to stay at Ayodhya to look after the kingdom in his absence. Fourteen years' of exile from a kingly abode, to live in thick jungles, specially bare-feet and with minimum clothes to wear, was a bad and long period for any one. Rama came back home only after completing fourteen years in the forests. It is said that Rama was an incarnation of Vishnu (Brahman). So he willingly suffered the pangs of life as an example to others just as Christ did. Whatever the case may be, the legends say that he was born just as a human being and lived and died like any other person. But he lived an unparalleled moral life though full of misery and unusual discomfort. It is because of that that in every small or big town in India as well as in the principal cities of the developed countries of the world, people have built Rama's temples. There, the statues of Rama, Sita and Laxman, have been installed. Rama did not preach any religion or formulated any moral code. But *Ramleela,* the story of Rama's life, is enacted on the stage in small or big towns in India and many countries of the world during a particular time of the year. Rama is remembered on account of his leading a pure and ethical life. He is, therefore also known as *Marayada Purushottom,* that means *One who always abided by the moral code.* Who made that code for him is not known to us. Perhaps he knew that the only meaning of life was to stay tuned with one's soul that is divine in nature. *So, Rama is immortal just like Buddha and Christ and will be remembered until the world lives.*[15]

Embodiment of Love

Except Buddha and Rama, no other human being has been more adored and respected in this world than the Christ. He not only loved his fellow beings but cared even for his enemies, and sacrificed his life for the love of his people and his beliefs that he reckoned true. In that respect we find some similarities between the lives of Jesus and Socrates. Both were born in the carpenters' families. Both persons were teachers of great distinction yet did not leave any writings of their own. Both conducted their teachings by means of conversations with individuals and were critical of the political and religious leaders of their time. Both proclaimed by their example a standard of moral conduct that was above the prevailing conduct of the recognized leaders of the society in which they lived. Both of them suffered a martyr's death and in some sense each of them arose from the dead and became immortal as their teachings and sacrifices made them alive and more powerful after their death.[16]

Jesus of Nazareth grew to manhood in a humble carpenter's home. He participated in all duties of his father's vocation, but also pondered deeply about the moral and religious needs of his people. His family was quite aware of the prevalent sectarian traditions and faith. But he did not show any inclination towards them, except that once, when on a trip to Jerusalem, the parents lost him when he was only twelve. They found him in the Temple, listening to the teachers and asking questions eagerly. Except for this incidence, nothing much of that nature has been reported of Christ. When he grew up very matured, he went to listen frequently to John's preaching. John's preaching was his first serious exposure to give birth to his faith to which he remained united until his death. He started believing that John was right and the Kingdom of Heaven was not far away if he could transcend himself spiritually. This sort of preparation must be deep and intense and affect his whole life. So he accepted baptism by John. As he was emerging from the water, he felt as if a deep sense of God's grace had dawned on him. That vision or strong feeling created a significant influence on him. Soon after that, he retired to the forest to ponder over the ideas that he had gathered in the company of the prophet, John. It gave him the opportunity to compare his newly sprouting thoughts with that of John's. In that process his convictions and faith towards God grew stronger. He did not agree with John in certain matters. He abandoned the idea of becoming an ascetic as he pondered on the issues relating to God. He felt convinced that 'nature with all her bounty and beauty, is God's creation. It could be accepted gratefully and trusted joyfully. There was nothing in it that could be rejected as intrinsically evil.' He also did not like John's approach of making people come to him if they wanted to hear him. Jesus loved the ordinary people with whom he had toiled as a carpenter. He knew many of them who were too much oppressed with their daily routine. They often had to travel away from home. They would not care to know about the spiritual truth if they had no time for it. So Christ decided to carry the good news of God's early coming to the people. Therefore, in a much clearer language that could explain the spiritual meanings of the obscure religious terms, such as Kingdom of Heaven, Christ started his journey of preaching the people. He often sought them at the synagogues for he knew that only pious people who were eager to listen, would come there. So, he would often gather a group of close friends and disciples around him. At times they were only twelve in number, selected from humble toilers, like fishermen, artisans, and sometimes a tax collector too.

Christ started spreading his religious message to the people, assuring them of God's presence. He gradually felt that peace and happiness started growing in his own heart as it was reported to be growing in the hearts of the loyal people who fully accepted his teachings. Perceptibly, a new insight developed in him that was akin to the insight possessed by the prophets who had come before him. The meanings of the questions like, 'when the Kingdom of God would come?,' became transparent to him. The Kingdom of God was not coming visible, as he had thought earlier like his predecessors. The enlightened Jesus conceived a new meaning of it now. He thought that to behold that Kingdom man would need to prepare himself. So far as the man's heart is sincere and genuine, the Kingdom would lie in his own heart. That means, 'if any human's soul undergoes true repentance and is inwardly transformed from a state of disobedience to the state of trustful obedience towards God, and relinquishes selfish attitude to a spirit of love and friendliness towards all his fellows, so far he is concerned the Kingdom of God has come to him without waiting for future'. He is then in a position to realize the inner integrity and the spiritual brotherhood with others. Consequently, he would be in possession of complete joy, peace and happiness. He is already in the Kingdom of God. Nothing more needs to happen so far as his individual experience is concerned. Soon a kind of enlightenment dawned on Jesus by a clear understanding of the concepts contained in the *Old Testaments*. He found in himself a power that he had not anticipated. With that power he healed many sick and ailing persons. He started thinking that he was the promised Messiah. With his growing popularity, it was certain that the priesthood and others in authority would take it as a threat against them. Rest of the story is already known to us.

In our search to know the answer to our basic question, I would like to draw the attention of the reader towards Jesus' teachings. They convey his moral precepts and guide us to lead a life implicit with inward purity and righteousness. He conceived distinctly that:

In the moral life it is the intention that counts, not the mere deed; lustful desire is just as guilty as adultery, and is so judged by Him who sees the thoughts of the heart as easily as any outward act. One must become clean on the inside, not merely to an external view. The kingdom for which all longed is not an affair of worldly conquest and material prosperity; it comes within the heart of each individual, and the significance of its external manifestations is just that they render vivid the judgment passed upon each man in accordance with the true state of his inward self.[17]

Thus, Christ contended that if a person desires to possess the Kingdom of God, he would surely have it, provided he is clean inside. For that the basic virtues that he ought to possess are, sincerity, truthfulness, earnest devotion to God, justice, heartfelt commitment to right, friendliness and love. Besides, his spiritual inwardness should develop not by withdrawing from the world, but within the framework of the material world, that is God's own creation. To understand Christ's hopefulness for persons who long to possess Kingdom of God within them, let us read from the Sermon on the Mount. It commands:

Blessed are those who feel their spiritual need,
for the Kingdom of Heaven belongs to them!
Blessed are the mourners, for they will be consoled!
Blessed are the lowly, for they will possess the land!
Blessed are those who are hungry and thirsty
for uprightness, for they will be satisfied!
Blessed are the single-hearted, for they shall see God!
Blessed are the merciful, for they will be shown mercy!
Blessed are the pure in heart, for they will see God!
Blessed are the peacemakers, for they will be called God's sons![18]

There has not been any prophet or God's messenger who has taught the importance of love more than Christ. In the Sermon on the Mount, Jesus directs his views to clarify the implications of this (love) principle, emphasizing forgiveness, readiness in serving others, avoiding hasty judgment, and need of repentance and self-criticism. All these virtues culminate love that is the most predominant virtue in the heart of Christ. He believes that wholehearted love towards

God and brotherly love towards man was one of the supreme values. Love towards God would mean one's total willful submission to Him; love to a person must extend to all without exception. It will also mean special care and compassion for those who are poor, sick, weak or unjustly treated. Christ's love is not confined to the sick and poor. He extends it to enemies too. Most truly it was so. At the time of his crucification, he prayed to God to forgive them who had been unkind to him. There lays the difference between Socrates and Christ. Socrates reproaches his enemies by exposing them for their follies and biased judgment against him; Christ seeks God's forgiveness for his enemies. Socrates' is a wise person and his approach is intellectual. Christ reflects his total faith in love and seeks forgiveness for his enemies. Who would do so but only he who loves the humanity truly. Can a person sacrifice anything more than his own life without understanding its meaning truly? Certainly not. Christ surely understood the meaning of the Self. The moral precepts he propagated, precipitated from his divine soul that we all possess, but are unable to fathom.

Man of Steady Wisdom

We are not strictly adhering to a chronological order in discovering the past to understand the meaning to know thyself. I would therefore, like to deal with one of the wisest of persons of the ancient times. He has aroused man's attention once again towards his ethical notions in the late twentieth century. He is popularly known as Lord Krishna, whose Divine Song contains the theory of *Karma* or 'Karma Yoga'. The Karma Yoga, if followed, may enlighten a person to perform his duty and responsibilities even amidst the consistent turmoil and confusion prevailing profusely in human lives.

Instinctively, due to our ignorance motivated by our ego, we often act by the force of our ego-centric desires. An uncultivated person acts unthoughtfully, making his own life a sorrowful existence. He acts in the world to seek joy when propelled by the sensuous desires. Instead he earns for himself short-lived happiness, endless sorrows and mental impressions (*vasanas*). These *vasanas* create new fields of attractions through their free expressions in actions. It results in a non-stop vicious circle of ego-motivated actions that create further *vasanas,* stopping him from choosing a right path in action. This is the prelude to the theory of Karma, that Krishna unfolds in the third chapter of the *Shrimad Bhagvad Gita*. Krishna's disciple-friend Arjuna, who in a battle field, refuses to fight his enemies as they happen to be his relatives although they have cheated and acted dishonestly against him. Arjuna's mind is so much overwhelmed with sorrow that he is unable to decide to act in want of right decision. The second chapter of the Gita contains that Krishna tries to dispel Arjuna's doubts and prepares him to fight as it is the duty of a monarch to fight against the wrong doers. In the beginning, Krishna's viewpoint is not clear to Arjuna. He gradually pays more attention. Slowly he tries to understand the meaning of the right karma or right duty contained in the following most popular verse (mostly misunderstood by the people) of the *Gita*. Krishna says:

कर्मण्येवाधिकारस्ते मा फलेषु कदाचन।
मा कर्मफलहेतुर्भूर्मा ते संगोऽस्त्वकर्मणि॥ ४७॥

Action is one's duty but reward is not his concern. One has a right and duty to act but if he also expects reward as a result of that duty, it would not be correct as reward is not his right. At the same time one must act, because not acting would mean not discharging one's duty.[19]

Listening to it, Arjuna requests Krishna to enlighten him further on 'what the right path is' and 'how to perform right actions.' Considering that Arjuna is still suffering from delusion, Krishna explains him, 'how he should act rightly and attain the highest goal of life.' He states that:

लोकेऽस्मिन्द्विविधा निष्ठा पुरा प्रोक्ता मयानघ।
ज्ञानयोगेन सांख्यानां कर्मयोगेन योगिनाम्॥ ३॥

There are two-fold paths for action. One is the 'path of knowledge' of Sankhya, the other is the 'path of action' followed by the Yogins. To consider that the path of action (karma yoga) is competitive to the 'path of knowledge'(janana yoga) would mean understanding neither of them. They are complementary to each other. They need to be practised one after the other.[20]

Krishna explains the meaning of the verse further. He says that 'selfless activity gives a chance to the mind to exhaust many of its existing mental impressions (*vasanas*). Mind, thus purified, gains great flight and eternal poise. Then, it can steadily ascend to the subtler realms of meditation, and finally come to gain the experience of the transcendental Absolute.

Swami Chinmayananda contends that religious men who are fit for spiritual discipline, fall under two distinct categories: the active and the contemplative. Temperamentally, these two kinds of men fall very much apart. Therefore, prescribing for both of them one and the same technique for individual development, would mean to discourage one section and ignore its progress. Since the *Gita* is not merely a text-book related to Hinduism, it is a kind of Bible of humanity, contends Swami Chinmayananda. As such, in its universal application, it has to show methods of self-development. These methods must suit the mental and intellectual temperaments of both of these categories of people. Krishna, therefore, explains clearly that the two-fold path of self-development (realization) prescribed for the world, (the Path-of-Knowledge and the Path-of-Action) is meant for the meditative and the active aspects respectively from the very beginning of the creation. The Path-of-Action is a means to an end, not directly, but only as a preparation to the Path-of-Knowledge. When the Path-of-Knowledge is attained, it leads to the goal directly without any extraneous help. Krishna continues explaining:

न कर्मणामनारम्भान्नैकर्म्यं पुरुषोऽश्नुते ।
न च संन्यसनादेव सिद्धिं समधिगच्छति ॥ ४ ॥

Man does not reach 'actionlessness' by non-performance of actions; nor by mere renunciation he attains Perfection. How can he reach Perfection then? Swami Chinmayananda, explaining the implicit meaning in the verse, comments that, 'Since the Self is pure, everyone of us is also Perfect. It is due to our ignorance of this spiritual experience that we entertain in our intellect unending desires, each of them being our own intellect's attempt to fulfil itself. Is it not a fact that we desire things that are already with us in satisfying quantity? As the desire in us, so are our thoughts. Thoughts are (in a way) disturbances created in our mental zone by our desires. The texture and quality of our thoughts are directly conditioned and controlled by our desires every moment. Thus, thoughts, expressed in the form of outer world of objects, become man's actions. And actions are nothing but man's thoughts projected and expressed in the world.[21]

In this *'chain-of ignorance'* constituted of desires, thoughts and actions, each one of us is caught and bound. If we observe carefully, we will find that there are not many different factors but only one, the spiritual 'ignorance'. It does not permit us to perform right actions. We have already discussed that when our ignorance (*avidya*) functions in the intellect, it becomes itself as desires. The desires, functioning in the mental zone, express themselves as thoughts. Thoughts become as actions when they express themselves in the outer world. So if we define the Supreme as 'the experience beyond ignorance,' it would not be incorrect. Therefore, it is necessarily true that the (pure) Self is *"the State of desirelessness"* or *"the Condition of thoughtlessness"* or *"the Life of Actionlessness."*[22]

After the above explanations we come back to the same question, 'How can one get Perfection?' The *Gita* unfolds that by mere 'renunciation of action' (*Sanyas*), no one can attain Perfection. Running away from life is not the way to reach the highest goal of evolution. What is the right way then? Krishna very thoughtfully discloses the process. He says, 'One can get Perfection through right action only. It can be attempted by purification of the inner instrument (mind). If the inner instrument is purified, man's thoughts are purified. Then the seeker can walk the Path-of Knowledge to reach ultimately the spiritual destination of Self-rediscovery.' This is the technique of self- development and Perfection. Krishna goes on adding more about performing action. He says.[23]

न हि कश्चित्क्षणमपि जातु तिष्ठत्यकर्मकृत्।
कार्यते ह्यवशः कर्म सर्वः प्रकृतिजैर्गुणैः।। ५ ।।

The Verse says that Verily, none can ever remain, even for a moment, without performing action; for, every one is made to act helplessly, indeed, by the qualities born of Prakriti.

Swami Chinmayananda explains further the implicit meaning in the verse. He states that man is always agitated under the influence of the triple tendencies of Inactivity (*Sattva*), Activity (*Rajas*), and Inactivity *(Tamas)*. These tendencies are inherent. Even for a single moment he cannot remain totally inactive. Total inactivity is the character of utterly insentient matter. Even if one is physically at rest, mentally one is active all the time, except when he is in the state of deep sleep. So long as one is under the influence of these three mental tendencies (*gunas*), one is helplessly prompted to act. Therefore, not to act at all would tantamount to disobeying the laws of nature. We all know that it would bring about a cultural deterioration in ourselves.

Thus, the Gita advises man to act vigorously with right attitude of mind, so that he may avoid all internal waste of energy and learn to grow in himself. Right attitude of mind has been stressed by both, the Western and the Eastern philosophers. I have already referred to Buddha's viewpoint in this respect and will discuss it again when I talk of Buddha's 'eight-fold- path' in this chapter. It is so important for any man to understand clearly that the attitude of mind is solely responsible to make him act good or bad. It is because of that the Gita has laid much stress on it. The mind has a tendency to repeat its own thoughts. When a thought is repeated again and again, it creates a deepening impression in the mind. As a result, all thoughts arising in it afterwards, flow in that prepared direction. When once the direction of the flow is fixed in the mind, all external activities of the individual are influenced by this tendency. Thus, a mind that constantly meditates on sensuous pleasures, creates for itself an intense sensuous tendency and helplessly act in that direction. Therefore, it is so important for a person to possess the right mental attitude. Knowing it well, Krishna goes on admonishing Arjuna to think rightly and do his duty. In doing so, he must not have any attachment to the thoughts (feelings) that are not worthy to be thought of. This is what Krishna means by possessing 'a steady wisdom'. In the ninth Verse of the chapter on 'Karma Yoga', Krishna stresses the importance of 'sacrifice'. Swami Chinmayananda beautifully clarifies the meaning of the term 'sacrifice'. The followers of the Gita have often misunderstood its meaning. The Verse says:

> *The world is bound by action other than those performed 'for the sake of sacrifice'; do thou, therefore, O son of Kunti, perform action for that sake alone, free from all attachment.*[24]

The meaning implicit in the verse is that every action does not bring about bondage upon the doer. It is only unintelligent activities that thicken the impressions in the mind. Such impressions build successfully a strong wall between the ego-centre and the *Divine Spark* of Life in us. Thus, actions, motivated by ego-centric desires do not permit a single divine thought to penetrate into man and lead him to commit sins. It is therefore, all activities, other than the *Yajana*-activities (sacrifices), are bound to bring about *vasana*-bondage. The correct meaning of *Yajana* (sacrifice) in a wider sense is only 'a self-sacrificing action. It is undertaken in a spirit of self-dedication for the benefit of all.' Such an action cannot be self-degrading but brings self-liberation. The appropriate meaning of *Yajana* can be understood as any 'social, communal, national or any personal activity. It is undertaken by the individual to pour himself readily in a spirit of service and dedication. Only when people act in a spirit of co-operation and self-dedication, the community can get itself freed from poverty and sorrow. Such activities can only be undertaken in a spirit of loyalty towards Divinity as then the worker has no attachment towards the actions. Thus, the Gita always commands man to perform actions without attachment. By performing actions in this manner, will help him to attain the Supreme.[25]

The Gita strongly pleads that we all need to follow the practical method. While we work, we should remain unattached to our ego-centric and limited concept of the Self and enter into the battlefield of turmoil and sorrows like a champion. We can fight then for the noble and righteous cause against those who challenge righteousness, upholding the values of higher living.[26]

The term "fight" is to be understood as our individual fight with circumstances, in the silent battle of life. Thus the advice is not for Arjuna alone, but to all men who would like to live life fully and intelligently! In order to explain clearly to all this new interpretation of the Vedantic truth, Krishna said:

> *Those men who constantly practise this teaching of Mine, full of faith and without caviling, they too are freed from actions.*[27]

In the above verse the importance of 'faith' and 'caviling' has been stressed in relation to practising the right activity. Faith (*Sradha*) in Vedanta means the ability to digest mentally, and comprehend intellectually the full import of the advice given by the Saints and contained in the Scriptures. The truth is that without faith no activity is ever possible. Faith can also not grow where intellectual beliefs and commitments are not there. Similarly, without unnecessary criticism or caviling, any intellectual principles cannot be understood or appreciated. Extending the meaning of the words, they too are freed from actions, Swami Chinmayananda states: 'The immature students of the Gita are advised to understand the meaning of the term 'worklessness' that Krishna uses all of a sudden. He insists most of the time that man should act diligently and rightly. It is mainly due to our lack of adequate understanding of the meaning of the term and not that it actually means non-action."

Thus the Gita repeatedly insists that the 'Path-of-Work' lies through a process of elimination of desires in us. When our desires are eliminated, the work accomplished is the true divine action. In order to detach ourselves from our likes and dislikes, we must get rid of our false ego-centric vanities that create *vasanas*. When the mind is free from *vasanas*, it becomes non-existent of ego, and is capable to understand the truth. The underlying idea is that at all occasions a wise man should be a master of himself. Being free from attachments and acting in the midst of situations of life, one can attain the highest goal of life that is experiencing the Absolute Bliss. This is the state of a man who has steady wisdom like the Lord Krishna.

Most Illumined

The most enlightened, who taught self-discipline in order to gain liberation from the wheel of life and rebirth, was known as Gautama Buddha. He was born a prince of the Sakya clan at Kapilavastu in North India, around the first half of the 6th century BC. His family name was Gautama, and given name was Siddhartha. Few people make use of these names now. Just as Jesus of Nazareth became to devoted followers and to the later generations in the West—the Christ, so this philosophical pioneer of India in the later centuries come to be known as the Buddha.

Buddha's original teaching was not a religion but a system of self-discipline and self-deliverance. He offered a 'way' of overcoming the fetters of life as well as reformation that was both social and spiritual. Even though he was born as a prince in a noble family of the warrior caste, he did not approve of the caste system, still prevailing in India. We would not go into the details of his life-history as like Christ, he too is well known, world over. According to the Buddhist tradition, he went to the Deer Park at Banaras, immediately after his illumination. He preached his doctrines to his former fellow hermits. He expressed that there are Four Noble Truths, that if understood well, *Nirvana* could be attained.

The First Noble Truth states that there is suffering or frustration in human life. It comes from our difficulty in facing the basic fact of life, that everything around us is impermanent and transitory. All things arise and pass away, said the Buddha.[28]

Suffering arises whenever we resist the flow of life and try to stick to fixed forms that are *Maya,* whether they are things, people, ideas or events. The doctrine of impermanence also includes the notion that there is no ego, no self. The idea of a separate individual self is an illusion, just another form of *Maya. It* is simply an intellectual concept. It has no reality.

The Second Noble Truth is the cause of all suffering. It is clinging. It is a baseless grasping of life based on *avidya* or ignorance. An individual divides the perceived world into separate things and thus attempts to confine the reality in fixed categories, that are simply his mind's creation.

So long this impression continues, man is bound to experience frustration as the things of the world are transient and bound to change. As long as this view prevails, the vicious circle perpetuates further, giving birth to new images. Consequently, every action generates further actions. At this point the Buddha seems to be very much influenced by the Vedanta as similar ideas have been projected in the Gita. Krishna reflects akin views in relation to man's right conduct and unerroneous actions. This vicious circle is known as *Samsara* in Buddhism. It implies unending chain of birth and rebirth that is instrumented by the 'Law of Karma'.

The Third Noble Truth deals that suffering can be removed or ended and the vicious circle of *Samsara* and the bondage of karma can be transcended and the state of complete liberation *Nirvana* can be attained. In this state of *Nirvana* or liberation or the false notions of ***separate self*** disappear forever, and oneness of total life becomes constant sensation. Thus, *Nirvana* is the same as *Moksha* in Vedantic or Hindu philosophy. It means the state of awakening.

The Fourth Noble Truth, according to the Buddha, is

end of all suffering through practising the 'eight-fold path' that leads to self-development and state of Buddhahood.[29]

This path includes eight steps, or systematic requirements indicated as follows:

- Right understanding
- Right purpose or aspiration
- Right speech
- Right conduct
- Right vocation
- Right effort
- Right mindfulness
- Right concentration

I shall explain briefly this 'eight-fold path' to clarify the significance of each step. The first two requirements form the preliminary essentials. One is unable to make any serious start towards the goal without that. In the absence of right understanding of what the real problem of life is, the goal cannot be understood. Similarly without right aspiration towards the right goal, one would never know in what direction to go. The next three requirements are conditions necessary as they imply aspirant's sincerity, determination and strength of self-control in abiding by what he sees is right. No spiritual growth is possible if one does not possess self-discipline, basically to avoid moral confusion. If one cannot follow the basic rules of moral conduct, he cannot be expected to renounce impulsive gratification of sensuous desires. These desires often conflict with the more rigorous requirements of spiritual progress.

Without abandoning wrong modes of gaining one's livelihood,* he cannot achieve the goal. One who has faith in the Buddha, must not earn his livelihood by working in places like slaughterhouses. He would never realize power for spiritual growth if he earns his living there. Thus these three steps constitute one's strong determination in readiness towards his daily acts. In a way they help sustaining the moral foundation required for his ethical growth. The remaining three requirements turn our attention towards the goal of completed self-conquest. Right mindfulness is required to purge

---

* Refers to everyday struggles in life to gain livelihood & thereby coming in conflict with the main goal he is sincerely aspiring to achieve.

tanha (trishna) or thirst for sensuous desires. As one's (disciplined) awareness grows, by rejecting *tanha* in every form, he gains more in power of concentration. In order to reach the stage of right concentration or right meditation, one has to conquer the distractions. These distractions come to him by way of craving for the interesting objects around him. When right concentration is achieved by right mindfulness and right concentration, the wandering of the mind is controlled by itself. Gradually, man becomes free from every selfish craving. He can see steadily and absorb himself in meditation, completely identifying himself with the truth. With this step of concentration or meditation, the final goal is reached. He gets freedom from the vicious circle of birth and rebirth. It is the final stage of the Buddhahood. In fact the purpose in explaining the basic Buddhist concepts is not merely acquainting the reader with the Buddhist principles enumerated for the benefit of his disciples. It is mainly to highlight him with some purpose. It is, that though the Buddha rejected that there is any soul, he could not dispel the idea that something existed like a soul. He called it 'a stream of consciousness.'* He was also sure that by reaching the state of *Nirvana* that is equivalent to Vedantic *Moksha,* one could attain complete bliss. It is the main goal of almost each school of philosophy in the East and the West, with a very few exceptions like the *Charvakas.* They desired for the attainment of material and sensuous pleasures, perhaps because they believed that Reality is composed of Matter only. If *Nirvana* or the highest state of spiritual bliss is the only goal of life, it can be realized by abiding by the Eight-fold Path. Does it not mean that the Great Buddha must have understood the divine purpose of this life? He therefore, insisted that misery and confusion rampant in our lives, needed redemption by constantly practising the regulations prescribed by him.

Buddha's technique of discourse is very natural and fascinating. When we read his discourses held with the monks, we come quite close to his thought process relating to his ethical ideals. Once, when he was preaching five disciples, who sat there in his presence, four

---

* Buddha identified soul as 'stream of consciousness', perhaps because he did not want to identify it in line with the Vedantic tradition as he rejected the Traditions.

out of them, did not seem to be paying any heed to him. The fifth one, Ananda, who stood there fanning the Master, observing the behaviour of those persons said to him:

> "Lord, Thou art teaching the Truth to these men even as the voice of the thunder when the heavy rains are falling. Yet behold! they sit doing this and that ....Thy teaching elevate even through the skin and reacheth unto bones and marrow. How can it be that when Thou preachest the Law these men pay no heed thereto?"

The Master replied:

> "Ananda, such things as the Buddha, or The Law, or The Order of Brethren, though countless hundred thousand cycles of time have never been heard of by these beings. Therefore they cannot listen to this Law. In this round of births and deaths, whose beginning is incalculable, these beings have come to birth hearing only the talk of divers animals. They spend their time in song and dance, in places where men drink and gamble and the like. Thus they cannot listen to the Law".
> "But what, Lord, is the actual reason, the immediate cause why they cannot?," asked Ananda.

The Master replied:

> "Ananda, owing to hatred, owing to delusion, owing to lust, they cannot do so. There is no such fire as the fire of lust. It burns up creatures, nor even leaves any one behind.... But this one, who, sitting, hears the Law attentively, for many, many times successively, was a master of the Vedas a brahmana who could repeat the Sacred Texts. So now also he pays good heed unto my words."[30]

Buddha's teachings unfold that belief in the supernatural, which is beyond his acceptance. He understood clearly that a person's ultimate goal in his life should be to lead a moral life. The moral principles that he evolved after a lot of suffering, wandering, toil, frustration, reflections and meditation, are the outcome of his penetrating and intellectual eye. It made him see that suffering and dismay could be totally removed from our lives. Unending bliss can surely be attained by following those moral practices. In fact the Great Buddha understood the meaning of life very vividly. If he had not, we would have neither called him the Illumined, nor ever revered him.

Our discussion on the Buddhist approach to *Nirvana* and attainment of tranquillity would not be complete if we don't discuss the Zen philosophy. In spite of special character, Zen is purely Buddhist in its essence. Its aim is no other than that of the Buddha himself. The attainment of enlightenment is an experience in Zen. It is known as *satori*. Although attainment of enlightenment is the essence of all schools of Eastern philosophy, Zen is unique in that sense. It concentrates mainly on this experience and is not concerned with any further interpretations.

When the Chinese philosophical thought came in contact with the Buddhist beliefs and principles around the 1st century A.D., the Buddhist *Sutras* stimulated Chinese thinkers. They led them to interpret the Buddhist teachings in the light of their own philosophy. This gave birth to a new philosophical thought-stream in China. The pragmatic side of the Chinese thought responded to the impact of Buddhism by concentrating on its practical aspects. It developed them into a special kind of discipline known as Ch'an. Usually it means 'meditation'. Later on around A.D. 1200, Ch'an's philosophy eventually became popular in Japan and cultivated under the name Zen. It can be summarized in the following four lines.

A special transmission outside the scriptures,
Not founded upon words and letters,
Pointing directly to the human mind,
Seeing into one's nature and attaining Buddhahood.[31]

The perfection of Zen means to live one's everyday life naturally and spontaneously. When one of the Zen masters was asked to define Zen, he said, when hungry, eat, when tired sleep. Although it sounds simple and very clear, it is in fact, quite a difficult task. To regain the naturalness of our original nature, one would need a long training. It would lead him to spiritual attainments. Zen's emphasis is on naturalness and spontaneity that must have been added to it by Tao's thought. The basis of this thought and movement is strictly Buddhist. ***It is the belief in the perfection of our original nature.***

The realization and the process of enlightenment consist of *in becoming what we are from the very beginning*. It is also the path of unity of man with himself.

It would not be true to state that the ancients whose life-style and ethical notions we have briefly discussed above, are the only noteworthy metaphysical and religious figures in the world. These few have been reported in this small work as our purpose was to enumerate the most conspicuous ones who seem to have understood the meaning of life very vividly. They transcended the ethical and moral heights to such immeasurable length that they do not seem to have any parallel in that respect. Even after and before the Christ, there have been an array of names of distinguished people who shook the world with their religious and philosophical notions. They brought a great revolution in the church and improved religious practices as they thought that the old canons had grown too traditional and ritualistic.

Besides, in our search of finding out 'the meaning to know thyself' only a few could be reported. In our attempt in that respect we have enlisted only those few who are beyond any controversy. They are known and loved by a great number of people all over the world. Still if someone has been left out by my inadequate insight and limited vision, I seek forgiveness of them who feel offended that way.

Including the past and the present, there seem to be two very distinguished philosophers who have indicated that if a person wants to know the truth, he should start first from himself. That is, to know the entire truth around him, he wouldn't need to know anything more than himself. *That knowledge alone would reveal him the vistas of truth that he would not get even if he spends his whole life for it.* One of those persons who initiated the notion of 'Know Thyself,' was Socrates whom we have already discussed. The other one known as Jiddu Krishnamurti, is next in line. He is reported in the next chapter.

References

The Concept of Unity

1. Brihadaraynka Upanisad, 4.5.15.
2. Trilochan Singh, (*et al*), *The Sacred Writings of the Sikhs*, Introduction.
3. S.R. Luis Vas, *The Mind of Krishnamurti*, p. 231.
4. Edwin A Burtt, *Man Seeks the Divine*, p. 4.
5. Charla H. Petterson & Gary Cares, *Plato's Euthyphro, Apology, Crito & Phaedo*, pp. 7–8.

6. Cora Mason, *The Man Who Dared to Ask,* pp. 29–30.
7. Cora Mason, *The Man Who Dared to Ask,* pp. 159–160.
8. Cora Mason, *The Man Who Dared to Ask,* p. 161.
9. Fritjof Capra, *The Tao of Physics,* pp. 91–92.
10. Burtt, *Man Seeks the Divine,* p. 157.
11. Burtt, *Man Seeks the Divine,* p. 158.
12. Lin Yu-tang (ed), *The Wisdom of China and India,* p. 831.
13. Lin Yu-tang, *The Wisdom of China and India,* p. 849.
14. Burtt, *Man Seeks the Divine,* p. 168.
15. Tulsidas, *Shri Ramcharit Manas,* (condensed).
16. Patterson & Carey, *Plato's Euthyphro, Apology,* p. 5.
17. Burtt, *Man Seeks the Divine,* p. 376.
18. *Condensed from the Holy Bible,* 5.3–12, p. 1074.
19. S. Radhakrishnan, *Bhagwad Geeta,* Verse 47, p. 124.
20. Swami Chinmayananda, *The Bhagwad Geeta, Karm Yoga,* Chapter 3, pp. 8–9.
21. Chinmayananda, *Karma Yoga,* Verse 4, p. 11.
22. Chinmayananda, *Karma Yoga,* p. 12.
23. Chinmayananda, *Karma Yoga,* Verse 5, p. 13.
24. Chinmayananda, *Karma Yoga,* p. 19.
25. Chinmayananda, *Karma Yoga,* Verse 19, p. 34.
26. Chinmayananda, *Karma Yoga,* Verse 25, p. 44.
27. Chinmayananda, *Karma Yoga,* Verse 31, pp. 54–55.
28. J Mascaro (ed), *The Dhammapada,* p. 113.
29. Firtjof Capra, *The Tao of Physics,* pp. 84–85.
30. F.L. Woodward, (trans), *Buddhist Stories,* pp. 64–68.
31. Firtjof Capra, *The Tao of Physics, p. 109.*

Quest of Unity

Man who provided the Procedure

Krishnamurti did not embellish his philosophical notions with any *a priori.* He did not seem to be influenced by any hunches that often precipitate in the minds of the scientists before they create new inventions. His education was slight and that too was accomplished with great difficulty. Still for more than half a century he discussed subjects that often touch human heart through his lucid and analytical discourses. He expounded many questions of metaphysical nature in the most original way that he discovered entirely from his own life's experience.

The discovery of this man who was to become Lord Maitre, was made by a distinguished theosophist named Charles Leadbeater. Leadbeater was reputed to have possessed highly developed psychic and clairvoyant powers. One day in the spring of 1909, he saw a group of Indian children bathing on the beach at Adyar. Adyar is near Madras that is a big town situated in the south-east of India. When he made a close observation of the children, he discovered some remarkable thing. He remarked to a close friend that one of those children had a remarkable aura. It indicated that he would become a great spiritual teacher as well as an orator. On inquiry, Leadbeater came to know that the boy was one of the four sons of a poor brahmin widower named Naraniah. He had held a humble position at the Madras branch of the Theosophical Society. When Leadbeater spotted Jiddu, he was a weak and undernourished child. He was around fourteen in age.

Jiddu Krishnamurti was born on May 11, 1895 in the town of Madanapalle in Andhra Pradesh to Telugu speaking middleclass brahmin parents. When his mother, Sanjeeveamma, sensed that her baby was one day to become a great soul, she insisted on delivering the child in the *puja* (prayer) room of her house. It was normally against the orthodox Hindu custom, but she delivered the child in that room. As the baby was the eighth in the family, they named him after Lord Krishna.

Krishna's father later on moved to Madras and took up employment with the Theosophical Society. Eminent persons like Annie Besant and Bishop Leadbeater led the Society at that time. Basic to the tenets of Theosophical was the belief that Lord Maitrey, the World Teacher—Christ in the West and Buddha in the East—manifests himself time to time. As such, he was soon to take a human form. When Leadbeater saw that the boy had the most luminous aura, he proclaimed that he would be the future Messiah. Many people were surprised to learn that the boy besides weak in health, was dull witted too. He was often punished at school and sent out on veranda, where he would keep watching the trees and birds.[1] Soon after Leadbeater discovered the child, Mrs Annie Besant became his legal guardian. He along with his younger brother, Nitya, was taken to England to get education there after sometime. On the 11th and 12th January, 1910, he was 'First Initiated' in the ceremony organized by Leadbeater. He got thoroughly convinced of his own role in future when he was indoctrinated with Theosophy. Some of the key metaphysical themes that he developed later on, seem to be a strong reaction against the indoctrination done at the time of his initiation. In the year 1911, a global organization called the 'Order of the Star of the East' was formed in the Theosophical Society. The Order was to prepare the way for the coming of the 'World Teacher.' Krishnamurti was nominated as its first head and retained that position for several years. While he was pursuing his studies, he continued as the head of the Order of the Star and wrote regularly for the Order's magazine. He was now twenty six years old and had acquired good confidence and authority in his role of the 'World Teacher.' It is reported that in 1921 some 2,000 members of the Society attended a Congress in Paris at which Krishnamurti spoke. He astonished all present there by his clear grasp of the questions raised, and the firmness with which he controlled the discussions. This was the beginning of a career of the great philosopher, who attempted to set human beings free from their self-created chains of bondage.

Conditioning as a Barrier

Krishnamurti expounded his philosophical vision for almost half a century. His clear challenging concepts have now come to notice of millions of people both in the West and the East. In spite of his great influence created by his clarity of thought and an untraditional outlook, it seems that many people have not been able to take advantage of his ideas. They either don't have time to read him or possess any desire to know him. He provided convincing solutions to attain freedom by means of simple logic and depth of his thought. It is sad that such a great thinker has not been a world changer, as was thought of him by Annie Besant. Still he certainly remains a mighty original thinker and an influencer of the world in the later half of the 20th century.

He possessed a simple and unassuming demeanour and a clear vision to analyze human problems. He provided soothing solutions to them and induced a new generation to revolt against materialism in favour of a simple and spiritual way of life. In this respect his influence, probably, has been more profound than that of any other publicized gurus who have emerged in the East in the recent years. In a most simple and convincing language Krishnamurti reasserts the importance of the ancient precept "know thyself." He advises us to seek liberation by acquiring the right knowledge that is the 'knowledge of one's own self.' In that quest he provides a procedure that is unique and unparalleled. He believes only in one value, 'self-knowledge,' that according to him, is valid and effective both for the individual and for the society. Human Being as a whole is in danger without that knowledge. In turn the humanity is in danger too. Krishnamurti contends that group is never total but only an individual is universal for individual makes humanity. A group does not think. It holds ideas and opinions but it can hardly hold clarity. A group is simply the organization of ignorance and of irresponsibility. Its actions are often regressive. If a person is fully conscious, he is creative. To create is to see things as they are. Creation implies a new vision and a clear consciousness. A group does not have that vision nor consciousness.

Krishnamurti has mostly been known as anti-traditional. He

does not accept the glamorous past on the grounds that it leads to conditioning. The present should not be built on the past. It may never lead to creativity and to new discovery. He comments that searching for the fundamental values has so far been a task of the few only. The majority of those who lived within a particular civilization, whether Brahmanist, Buddhists, Christian or Jews, etc. felt relatively comfortable within their mental and physical state of conditioning. They did not feel themselves frustrated in their creativeness. They never cared whether they need to discover the real purpose of life. It is the reason that even if they were ignorant about the truth, it did not matter much for them. Therefore, those who feel the need to break their conditioning must creep into themselves silently. They should understand clearly that conditioning destroys the original and creative liberty of human being.

Krishnamurti contends that an individual is more in bondage now than he has ever been. This fact is quite obvious. More than acquiring freedom, human being is trying hard for his future security. He lives in fear of varied kind—fears that are often untrue and unfounded. But the truth is that 'to perceive what freedom is, and of what it is made up, is no longer a question of personal preference.' Rather 'it is a matter of life and death,' contends Krishnamurti. Therefore, we should direct our first efforts towards the immediate necessity for insight and clear understanding. That would help in breaking down the conditioning. Is it so easy to break down the conditioning that has come to us since our birth without notice?

Krishnamurti frankly states that it is difficult to break down the barriers because our thought is accustomed to function in a way that conditions it regularly. Our mind regards itself identified with an 'I'. This identification has become so permanent throughout its existence, that all seem to be the product of an automatic process. This process has sought to justify itself in every possible way, but more especially through the canons of religion. It has been going on ever since human being began to talk and hold discourses. This sort of conditioning can be removed if an individual tries hard, not physically but mentally. Let us examine how our minds can help us in that process of econditioning, which is paramount for our freedom and self-knowledge.

Way to Self-knowledge

Individual must, if he desires to see himself in reality, clear his mind to an unimaginable extent. Krishnamurti reflects:

> *To see ourselves exactly as we are is the truth. Let us not go any further nor anywhere else. To be aware of what is in our consciousness from day to day, from moment to moment, when faced with a life's challenge, is, by itself, knowledge, complete, infinite, timeless.*[2]

It is not so simple to have that kind of awareness and remove all the conditioning that Krishnamurti is indicating. The fact is that it is difficult to do so. Carlo Suars remarks that though truth is simple, but it is so complex that one cannot conceive it easily. The precept 'know thyself' has been reflected by the philosophers in different centuries. Therefore, nothing seems to be very new in this commandment. At the same time it seems rather doubtful also that 'self knowledge' can be the key to all our problems. Krishnamurti also does not mention that it would be a good thing if we know ourselves. Neither he expresses that to possess that knowledge would pacify or comfort our lives. Still it is very important as:

> *Self-knowledge is action, immediate, powerful, concrete, the only one which can bring us out of our state of confusion. It is as urgent, real and practical as leaping into a lifeboat at the time of a shipwreck.*[3]

The intellectuals or wise persons, who believe and feel the presence of a complete human crisis, will surely not fail to understand Krishnamurti's explanations of the precept 'know thyself'. Krishnamurti does not mean to shatter our inner world nor he desires us to lose our own identity. The implications of the meaning of the 'precept' are vast and profound. To understand all about it one must reach it with a still and tranquil mind. Only then its meaning will brighten up with a secret and profound clarity. First of all, it reveals that no one can know us but ourselves. And that, since we are, all of us, the result of the past, by understanding ourselves we shall discover all knowledge, all wisdom.[4] In that process of knowing ourselves, our consciousness is obviously the best instrument to examine us from within. It can never fully examine others as it cannot enter others' interior. When we examine us from within, we find that the life within us is actual, present and active. This is what Krishnamurti believes. It is the cause of its past, that is an accumulation of struggles, reactions, hidden desires, losses of money and individuals, defeats and humiliations. When all that is discovered, it would cease to be the past. With that knowledge we shall discover 'what secret motive, what mysterious urge has led us to identify itself with an 'I am'. When these thoughts will come to our life—to our conscious self as we go on meditating, we will need no answers to many of those urges. Most of them are simply our reactions to certain motives. Then we shall be able to see deeper into us and will understand ourselves better, provided we do not implicate ourselves with that process of uncovering our past.

Through that process our mind will reveal ourselves from within. Our emotions, our feelings, perceptions and sensations, our dreams and the symbols that have meaning in life, will come to surface. Our conscious and unconscious worlds, that are more authentically our substance than our ideas and opinions, will be revealed before us. To see all that as it is, we would need 'to strengthen in us the state of our mind.' Only with that kind of mental state we would be able to develop keen observation and intense awareness. It would make us impartial, disinterested and simple like a storekeeper looking after the registering of swift coming and going of goods. Such storekeeper would lose his efficiency if he wasted his time in contemplating the objects, in criticizing them, in chatting about them. If he is absent minded, the traffic will escape him.[5]

Without that state of mind that is fully alert and aware, one would never be able to register every feeling correctly. He would also not be able to know himself completely. The process to the knowledge of the self, that Krishnamurti advises us to keep going, is not very simple, though most beautifully and logically he explains all its implications. He believes that the act of knowledge is immediate, being observation of what is.

As the individual goes on exploring he discovers that his problems and ardent desires are due to his way of thinking and feelings. Problems crop up on account of his belonging to a group, class, religion or a nation. Krishnamurti reminds us that most of family tragedies are due to the fact that we identify ourselves with traditional and collective ways of behaviour. When tragedies are provoked by habits and customs that are alien to us, they seem very big and unbearable. When they are dominated by religion, they become still bigger. Then we ask the religious authorities of our faith to solve those problems that they themselves have created for us. Is it not true that by doing so we are claiming to cure evil by evil? The truth is that no one can enlighten a person about the secret meaning of a reaction, a fleeting emotion or the hidden thoughts that constitute his substance every day all the time. No one can find meaning of his inward self that constantly live with him. If that is so, is it then necessary to follow the advice of the wise people from the past, when the causes of one's troubles are hidden in himself? Thus, in trying to understand the knowledge of ourselves, we find answers to most of our problems. We also come to know that the individual problem is also social and the social is also individual. It is really not possible to know ourselves without knowing our relationship with the world and persons with whom we live every day. So if we desire to know ourselves as we really are, it can be through our contacts and our conflicts. Therefore, Krishnamurti rejects any idea of isolating ourselves by meditating on self-knowledge. That kind of separation would mean a reaction against our problems and would never reveal to us our true self. The isolation in any case would be an illusion, because relationships would still stay within us, however, ignorant we play about them.

We should thus try to reach a state of balance, of serenity, and of contemplation, if we wish to possess self-knowledge. Even to seek God or truth, is to seek *not* to know ourselves, remarks Krishnamurti. If we only seek material security, it would finally end up one day in rediscovering both insecurity and life. Thus, man's primary duty is not to behave like a blind person, but to discover himself. For that he need not to 'believe' that he has an immortal soul or whether God or soul exists or not. All those kinds of beliefs really lead us no where. The important thing is that one should feel totally, not partly, responsible for possessing knowledge of oneself. This knowledge in itself is a unique value, both individually and collectively as human being always lives with some kind of relationship. This kind of integration will make man look vividly and will stop him from getting spilt up into pieces. Krishnamurti thus points out that if an individual is desirous to possess 'self-knowledge', he ought to be free from every kind of conditioning. Beliefs that one belongs to the East or to the West, are meaningless. Whether the spirit is real or matter is less real, are simply man's own reactions triggered off by his conditioning. Self-knowledge is the only knowledge that opens a new world for us. In that new world our being would stay undivided and integrate into one whole, totally united and devoid of conditioning or preconceived notions. Such notions simply create divisions between self and the Self.

Thus, Krishnamurti presents some unusual thoughts that are not common to many of us. The truth is that we do not see things as he does. He states that if a person accepts the precept 'self-knowledge,' it will be valuable. He will then discard all beliefs, all tradition, all the sacred scriptures of the East and the West. He will reject all interpretations made by individual and the world, and condemn all ideologies and even all ways of thinking. In that process of emptying the mind from all what has been taught, only a fresh and simple mind will evolve. It will then be able to see 'what is'.[6]

Self-knowledge leads to Freedom

Krishnamurti believes that the process of freedom begins with the 'choiceless awareness' of what one wills as well as of one's reactions to the symbol-system that tells one that one ought, or ought not to will. Through the choiceless awareness when one penetrates the successive layers of ego and its associated sub-conscious, love and understanding come. Krishnamurti reckons that this choiceless awareness at every moment and in all the circumstances of life is the only effective meditation. Except the state of choiceless awareness of mind, there is no other form of *samadhi* or *yoga,* that would show a person the path to liberation. It is the only state of mind in which it does not force itself to see the usual patterns backed by its beliefs and preconditioning. Aldous Huxley elaborating Krishnamurti's vision of liberation states:

> *True liberation is 'an inner freedom of creative Reality'. This is not a gift; it is to be discovered and experienced. It is an acquisition to be gathered to yourself to glorify yourself. It is a state of being, as silence, in which there is completeness.* [7]

The inner freedom can bring creativity and provide the vision of truth. It can come through the choiceless awareness that is also a prerequisite to self-knowledge. This kind of freedom is neither a gift nor an outcome of talent. It is to be found where thought frees itself from lust, ill-will and ignorance as well as frees itself from worldliness and personal cravings. It can only be experienced through right meditation. In other words it is choiceless awareness.

Commenting on Krishnamurti's unusual power of analyzing human problems and his originality of thought, Leonard Sainville, the famous author of the prize winning novel, *Dominique, the Negro Slave*, writes:

> *I admire his ability to state clearly certain problems. I am also quite willing to admit his absolute disinterestedness. And I admire what is most original in him—his desire to make us think for ourselves, in defiance of all dogmatic authority.*[8]

It is beyond doubt that Krishnamurti was a person of great talent. He possessed unusual insight with which he could analyze severe human problems and provide solutions to them. It was the reason that ailing minds often visited him to seek solutions to their problems and to understand the nature of truth as well. In the latter half of the twentieth century there is hardly any philosopher of his stature who possessed as much depth and clarity of thought as he did. He is the one who had refocused the issue of conditioning and showed the importance of the precept 'know thyself.' Like Socrates and Confucius he too saw all human problems originating from the individual. Therefore, his belief that the knowledge of the self is a value in itself, is surely of great importance. It can surely lead to unending vistas of truth and perpetual happiness.

Retrospective Reckoning

There is a saying in one of the Indian languages that 'only a few fully bloomed flowers are worthy to be offered at the God's altar.' That means not all fully bloomed flowers are picked up by the priest for the offerings. Only those that have fragrance and that look good, are accepted for the altar. In the same manner only those persons, who have fragrance of goodness and truthfulness, are beautiful. They are worthy of reverence and love. We all want to be loved and respected. But most of us do not know that without becoming good, it is rather impossible to get love or respect. Socrates was not much educated but he had the power to see things clearly. At an early age he discovered that the goodness in things makes them beautiful and useful. Knowing it is very important said Socrates. The Christ knew that if a person wanted to possess the Kingdom of God, he would surely have it provided he is clean inside. He said, 'Blessed are those who feel their spiritual need, for the Kingdom of Heaven belongs to them.' Rama had to lead a life that was full of extreme hardships. He always abided by the moral precepts, that made Him see upright and do 'good' only. Krishna invoked Arjuna to do his duty in accordance with the 'law of karma'. It was nothing else than to discharge one's duty strictly in line with the code of conduct prescribed for each individual in whatever vocation he may be. He knew it that if a person sought rewards in return of his duty, he would never be able to discharge his duty completely. Confucius knew very thoroughly that 'one should not do to others what he does not wish them to do to him.' He knew that the truth by which a person can live whatever the circumstance into which he may fall, is the truth that he discovers from within through his insight. It is the truth that is in tune with the way of Heaven. That truth would surely overcome his anxiety and fear. The enlightened Buddha discovered 'eight-fold path' that would lead his disciples towards *Nirvana,* that is a complete blissful state of mind. Each one of these persons, including Jiddu Krishnamurti, discovered that freedom and eternal bliss could be attained if a person knew that the right meaning of this life was to stay good. That means he should lead life in accordance with the precepts implicit within himself. No one can see correctly if he forgets that true meaning of this life is to act rightly and to live in accordance with good. To learn it that good lies within him, he does not need to go anywhere else but to discover his own self. That was the reason that Jiddu Krishnamurti and Socrates considered the precept so valuable. That was the only reason that most distinguished persons in different centuries and different countries, whether inspired by religion, politics or love, knew it well.

Why are we here?

Why we all are here is the question we need to ask ourselves every time. Somehow we all get it mixed up. We seem to be convinced that the real purpose of life is to try and outdo everyone else. It is to chase endlessly after goals that always help us slip away from unhappiness and misery. Consequently, we see people pushing, striving, worrying and making life a game of acquiring possessions or attaining high social positions. Most of us forget that inner satisfaction is the only goal worthy to chase.

Wayne Dyer comments that 'the purpose of this life in the modern society appears to be setting future-oriented goals. Some of these are—pleasing our parents or getting good grades on report cards, diplomas from the 'right' universities, job titles and promotions, awards, money, cars and televisions, etc.[9] We all seem to be so busy in chasing after external objects that we have no time for enjoying ourselves or to see the right purpose of life. If once we would put the question to ourselves 'Why are we here?', perhaps we would not wander in quandary.

The truth is that a few people ask that question to themselves. Therefore, only few know its meaning. Even if someone thinks that the purpose of life is only enjoyment, he should also know that enjoyment is not accomplished at the cost of others. Exploitation and fulfilment of one's desires in that manner, would never lead to a lasting happiness. If it were not true, neither Gandhi, Martin Luther, Martin Luther King, nor Abraham Lincoln would have given their lives for others. They knew it well that life has other meanings too. It included love and care for others. If Socrates did not have any love for the truth, he would not have given his precious life for the sake of it. Christ's example in that respect is surely unparalleled.

Perhaps, either on account of the objective attractions that lurk around us all the time, or on account of our endless desires originating from every kind of lust, we forget the real goal of life. In order to seek that goal, Krishnamurti asks us to look into ourselves with an alert and attentive mind devoid of conditioning. The procedure suggested by him appears to be quite simple. It does not demand us to practise it regularly. By looking at things correctly means cultivating a vision that is free from beliefs, religious prejudices, lust and attachment to the tradition. Is it really so simple to do so? Are there some real and simple procedures to follow what is 'good' and to see it distinctly so that most of our problems are solved at the very inception? Let us reflect on it and discover some possible ways that can help elevate us and make us see more clearly.

Some Possible Procedures

One of our crucial problems is transcending ourselves from the basement to the top story of our building where more light and air are available. This problem has become more acute as we don't have much time for us. Therefore, our sight and dimension of vision have gradually decreased on account of our constantly living in the basements of our lives. I recall a small incident that took place at the time when I was in the final year of high school, studying in my home town. The east-side of the school building that had four stories, was closed for the students on account of safety reasons. We had also been told that a few years back a student fell off from the top of the fourth story and died. Since then those rooms were used as store rooms. They were opened only when required. Once when the school physical instructor, who was quite friendly, opened the lock of the entrance to those rooms, I requested him to take me to the top of the building. After a while he agreed to take me there. When I reached the top, I was amazed to see the spectacular sight that presented a different picture of the small town. It looked so beautiful—all green and fascinating. I could see the whole town from the top. I had never been to that height in my life before. It was altogether a different sight that I could never imagine. Is it possible to see ourselves in a similar vein by removing our short-sightedness that is often imposed on us by our selfish inclinations, prejudices and unfounded fears?

Perhaps it may be possible. What we really need is to stop for a while from our daily routine and devote a few minutes to self-reflection. It will surely provide new visions and help us understand our prejudices and impulsive behaviour toward others. We do not forgive people until we don't understand that many a time it is 'me' who is the main cause of the trouble. Forgiveness is such a virtue that besides bringing the opposite poles together, it also *elevates* a person to a height he has not visited before. Forgiveness is often related with one's anger. No one can forgive others unless he spits his anger. In the second chapter of the *Gita,* Shri Krishna tells Arjuna that anger destroys man's intellect and consequently his wisdom too. When one is in rage, his power of discriminating right from wrong disappears. The most simple way to reduce the angry mood is to remove the self from the scene and stop thinking on the issue for a moment. It will certainly help toning down the mood. It looks so simple that many of us would surely say 'Oh, I know it.' How many of us really try it? These are very simple ways to stop one from falling down further.

Connected with the above thought-process is the right-mindfulness. The great Buddha also suggested something similar. Among his 'eight-fold path', right-mindfulness is one. Well, I am not promising anyone to attain *Nirvana.* I am certainly indicating that *right-mindfulness* is a process to transport a person from the lower story of his mental level to a much higher one, where from he can see light and experience happiness. I am quoting a beautiful example from a talk delivered at Sri Aurobindo *ashram* (a place for religious gathering) at Poona, India. 'A man is sitting in the fifth-storey of a building, contemplating on an important issue. That building has six stories. The last one is half done and is open to the sky. He has hardly concentrated for a few minutes that some guests arrive. He chats with the guests for a while and gets down to the ground floor to see them off. It is only after sometime that he remembers that he has something important to contemplate. He comes back again to the fifth storey. It happens each day and he never gets time to visit the last storey to see the light and enjoy the fresh air. The guests' visiting is so regular and frequent that he has no time to visit the open air space of his building.'

Perhaps, it happens with us quite frequently each day. When we start thinking in the right direction, our thoughts get distracted by the nasty ideas (guests) that we hardly keep going with the useful ones. Is it not feasible for us to adhere to the good thoughts, so that they carry us to the right direction? It is possible only when we have right-concentration. It also means *right-mindfulness.*

If we try to observe our thought-process from a distance, we will find that they become instrumental in making us indulge in various moods. For example, when one is in a doleful mood, thoughts of that nature constantly invade him, indulging him further in the same direction. Similarly, good and happy thoughts too create their impact on man's moods. Jiddu Krishnamurti has thrown much light on it. He indicates that 'thought' is a barrier to our freedom. Therefore, it is imperative to have *right-mindfulness.*

A few more things need to be added here. They are related to our thinking process. How often we go on condemning, comparing and identifying things which really don't have much importance in our lives! Perhaps, it goes on each day for a considerably long period of time. It would not be true to say that all the time we remain indulged with these three 'villainous thoughts,' but we do indulge with them often. Is it possible to get rid of such monstrous thoughts and save us from displeasure, hatred, anguish, fear and disharmony? If we can do it, we will not only be free from hatred, anger and disharmony, but will also enjoy our daily routine and see things clearly by staying united with ourselves. Let me briefly elaborate the terms *condemnation, comparison* and *identification.*

Unfortunately, on account of our short-sightedness and personal prejudices we start disliking our neighbours, friends and relatives. They often become targets of our criticism during our daily conversation. It provides us a kind of satisfaction and short-lived pleasure that normally we don't get from other kind of conversation. As a result, we go on *condemning* our friends and relatives without any reason, and go on enjoying queer satisfaction out of our self-justification. It gives birth to another nasty thought—*comparison.* It may also happen the other way too. The habit of constantly *comparing* ourselves with others in terms of money, personal achievements, material goods, such as the size and quality of television or car, may lead us *condemning* the people whom we are comparing with us. Thus, *comparison* and *condemnation* go hand in hand and constantly disturb our minds without the knowledge of the people whom we are criticizing or comparing. It gradually pulls us down to our basements, leaving a bitter taste in our mouths. This sort of involvement first starts during our talks. Then it drags us to act against the people who are totally unaware about the situation. This vicious circle goes on and on until we are trapped in some kind of difficulty. It could have been averted easily if we were not involved in *comparison* and *criticism.*

Let me explain *identification* with a few some examples. It so happened once when a rich person returned from a long tour, his neighburs informed him that his big house, near the lake, had caught fire and was burning. The rich person ran to the site and started crying at the sight of the burning house. In the meantime his eldest son, who had also reached there, told him that he should not cry. Before he had left for the tour, he had already made a deal to sell that house. The son also informed the wailing father that the person who had promised to buy the house, was a good person and would never refuse to pay even though the house got burnt. Listening to his son's conversation the rich person stopped crying. The thought that 'the burning house did not belong to him' made him free from identifying the house as his own.

Like the rich person, we all go on having unusual attachment towards the objects, relatives and even 'thoughts.' This sort of indulgence is likely to create problems for us. Can we remove *identification* from our minds and feel free from getting involved with the matters that don't need our attachment? We do need to love our children and other members of family, but extreme identification will surely lead to many sorts of problems. One of them is that when we lose any one of the loved ones, we can hardly tolerate it and plunge into dismay. Love implies duty. It implies commitment. If one discharges his duty without any expectations as the *Gita* has advised us, perhaps the intensity of identification may get reduced.

Well, getting rid of the nasty ideas, such as comparison, condemnation and identification, may help us to some extent. But we must keep track of our thoughts and divert them to right direction. Without it we cannot transcend ourselves to a higher plane. This entire life is a kind of game in which the player is the mind. How does one take advantage of one's mind, is a matter of great importance for each one of us. We all fail at some occasions, but we don't fail every time. Some may assign it (winning and losing) to one's luck, but I reckon that the proper use of one's mind, can surely help diverting catastrophes. Socrates used his mind by constantly asking questions and thus reaching the truth. Confucius devised the 'Golden Rule' that placed him as one of the best intellectuals China has ever produced. Shri Krishna visualized that 'Karma-yoga' was the best procedure to act in this world. The Christ gave up his life as for him 'love' was the highest virtue. Shri Rama led an unparalleled life that was in line with the highest code of conduct. The Great Buddha acquired the wisdom to enlighten the posterity with the procedure that could mitigate misery and reduce unhappiness in man's life. Krishnamurti discovered metaphysically an easy procedure to know the Self. All these great persons understood the meaning of their lives correctly and tried very hard to remain united with their own Self. In that process of seeking unity, they always used their minds in the best possible ways. Therefore, *right-mindfulness* is of supreme importance for each individual. It would provide him an opportunity for self-reflection and self-correction. At the same time it will help him to practise right-concentration and elevate him from his baseness that creeps into him on account of his ignorance *(avidya)*. It *(avidya)* has been a great concern of the philosophers in the East and the West. How can a person understand the meaning of his life when he is not conscious of using the mind for his own good! Those who know to use it well, they also know the true meaning of their lives. For such men, life is more meaningful as they live in unity with it.

References

The Quest of Unity

1. Krishna K. Murti, "J. Krishnamurti: The Solitary Pilgrim," *The Indian Express*, 28th Feb. ,1986, p. 8.
2. Carlo Suares, (trns.), *Krishnamurti And The Unity of Man*, p. 7.
3. Carlo Suares, *Krishnamurti And Unity of Man*, p. 8.
4. Carlo Suares, *Krishnamurti And Unity of Man*, p. 9.
5. Carlo Saures, *Krishnamurti And Unity of man*, p. 10.
6. Carlo Saures, *Krishnamurti And Unity of Man*, pp. 12–18.
7. Aldous Huxley, Forward to, *The First And Last Freedom*, p. 17.
8. Cited by Andre Nell, *The Man in Revolt*, p. 78.
9. Wayne Dyer, *The Sky's The Limit*, p. 40.

Bibliography

1. Banerjee Nikunja Vihari, (1973), *Philosophical Reconstruction,* New Delhi: Arnold-Heinemann India.
2. Burtt Edwin A., (1957), *Man Seeks the Divine,* New York: Harper and Brothers.
3. Capra Fritjof, (1976), *The Tao's Physics,* New York: Bantam Books.
4. Durant Will, (1970), *The Story of Philosophy,* New York Washington Sq. Press.
5. Chatterjee S.C. & Dutta D, *An Introduction to Indian Philosophy,* Calcutta: University of Calcutta., India.
6. Davids, C. Rhy, (1977), *Dialogues of the Buddha,* Sacred Books of the Buddhistic Series, (trans) by T.W. Davids & C.A. Davids, Republished by Motilal Banarasidas, S. Asia.
7. Dyer Wayne, (1980), *The Sky's The Limit,* New York: Simon And Schuster.
8. Fingsten Peter, (1956), *East Is East,* Philadelphia: Muhlenbarg Press.
9. Hiriyanna M, (1951), *Outlines of Indian Philosophy,* London: George Allen & Unwin.
10. Hiriyanna M, (1949), *The Essentials of Indian Philosophy,* London: George Allen & Unwin.
11. Holroyd Stuart, (1980), *The Quest of the Quiet Mind,* Northamptonshire: The Acquarian Press.
12. Hume David, (1978), *Treatise on Human Nature, Book I, (ed),* Selby-Bigge L.A. & Nidditch Peter H, Paper back.
13. Krishnamurti Jiddu, (1969), *Freedom From The Known, (ed)* Mary Lutyens, New York: Harper and Row, Publishers.
14. Krishnamurti Jiddu, (1969) *Freedom From The Known* (ed) Mary Lutyens, New York: Harper and Row, Publishers.
15. Luis Vas, (1971), *The Mind of Krishnamurti,* Bombay: Jaco Publishing House.
16. Loomis L.R., (1943), Aristotle: *On Man In The Universe,* (ed), New York: Walter J Black.
17. Lin Yu-tang, (ed) (1942), *The Wisdom of China and India,* New York.
18. Mascro J, (ed) (1973) *The Dhammpada,* Baltimore: Penguin Books.
19. Mason Cora, (1953), *Socrates: The Man Who Dared to Ask,* Boston: The Beacon Press.

20. Moore Charles A., (1951), *Essays in East-West Philosophy*, Honolulu: University of Hawaii Press.
21. Moore G.E., (1953), *Lectures on Philosophy*, (ed), Casimir Lewy, London: George Allen & Unwin Ltd.
22. Marias Julian, (1967) *History of Philosophy*, New York: Dover Publications Inc.
23. Patrick G.T.W., (1952), *Introduction to Philosophy*, Boston: Houghton Mifflin Co.
24. Petterson C.H. & Gary Cares, (1975) *Plato's Euthyphro, Crito & Phaedo*, Lincoln: Nebreska.
25. Radhakrishnan S., (ed) (953), *History of Philosophy, East and West*, Vol.-II, London: George Allen & Unwin Ltd.
26. Radhakrishnan S., *Bhagwad Geeta*, Delhi: Rajpal & Sons. (Hindi Version).
27. Rajneesh Acharya, (1984), *The Rajneesh Bible*, Vol. I, Oregon: Rajneesh Foundations Internationals.
28. Rajneesh Acharya, (1985), *The Rajneesh Bible*, Vol. II, Colorado: Rajneesh Publications Inc.
29. Rajneesh Acharya, (1985), *The Rajneesh Bible*, Vol. III, Oregon: Rajneesh Foundations International Rajneeshpuram.
30. Swami Chinmayananda, (1991), *The Karama Yoga, (The Bhagvad-Geeta)*, Bombay: Central Chinmaya Mission Trust.
31. Swami Prabhupada, (1975), *Bhagwad Geeta As It Is*, New York, Bhaktiveddanta Book Trust.
32. Swami Swarupananda, (1967), *Shrimad Bhagvad Gita*, Calcutta: Advait Ashram.
33. Sharma R.N., (1972), *Indian Philosophy*, New Delhi: Orient Long Man.
34. Stumpf S.E., (1971), *Philosophical Problems*, New York: McGraw Hill Book Co.
35. Strawson P.F. (1968), *Studies in the Philosophy of Thought and Action*, London: Oxford University Press.
36. Suares Carlo, (1973), *Krishnamurti And The Unity Of Man*, Bombay: Chetana Private Ltd.
37. Thilly Frank, (1953), *A History of Philosophy*, (rev. Ladger Wood), New York: Henry Holt and Co.
38. Tulsidas, (1939), *Shri Ramcharit Manas*, Gorakhpur, Geeta Press, U.P., India, (Hindi).
39. Warren H.C., (1934), *Buddhism in Translation*, Harvard University Press. Reprinted, (1995), Motilal Banarasidas, S. Asis.
40. Woodward F.L., (Trans) (1925), *Buddhist Stories*, Madras: Theosophical Publication House.
41. Wolfson Harry Austryn, (1973), *Studies in the History of Philosophy and Religion*, Massachusetts: Harvard University Press.
42. Windelband W., (1954) *A History of Philosophy*, (trans), James H. Tufts, New York: The MacMillan and Co.
43. *The Holy Bible, (1970)*, New Jersey: Thomas Nelson Inc.

GENERAL HEALTH

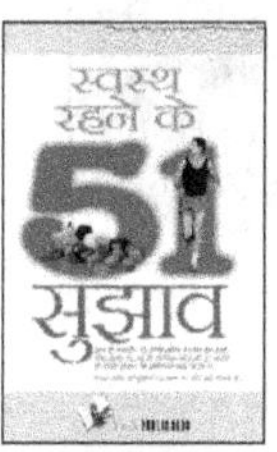
163 pp • ₹ 80

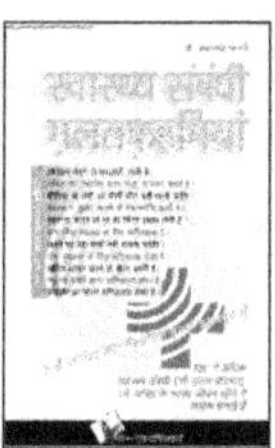
180 pp • ₹ 96

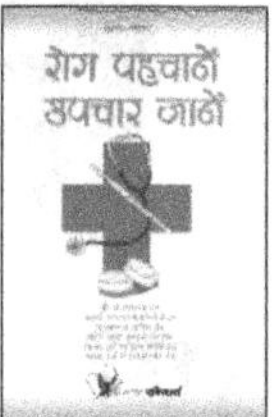
198 pp • ₹ 80

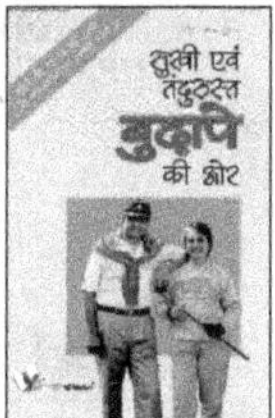
144 pp • ₹ 48

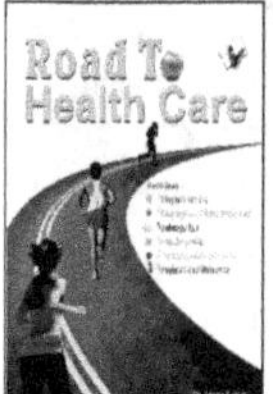
176 pp • ₹ 175

ALTERNATIVE THERAPIES

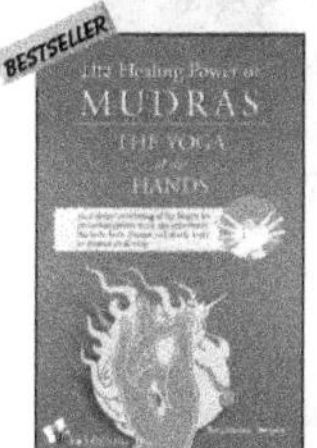
104 pp • ₹ 96

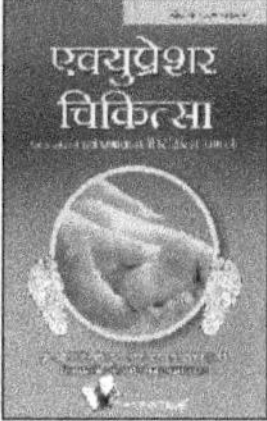
144 pp • ₹ 80

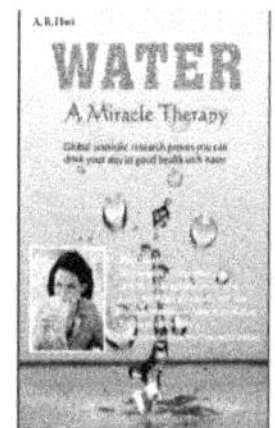
112 pp • ₹ 80

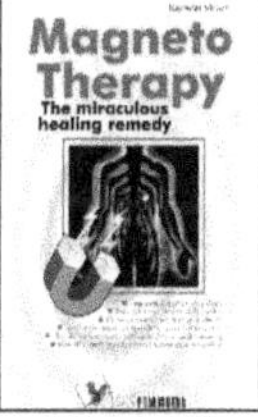
125 pp • ₹ 108

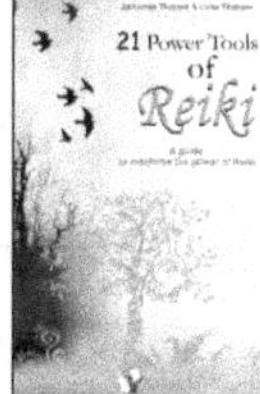
135 pp • ₹ 108

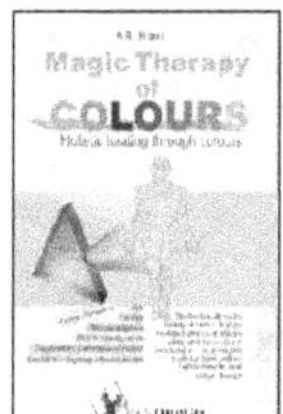
119 pp • ₹ 96

AYURVEDA

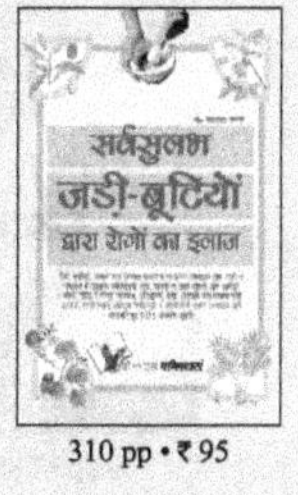
310 pp • ₹ 95

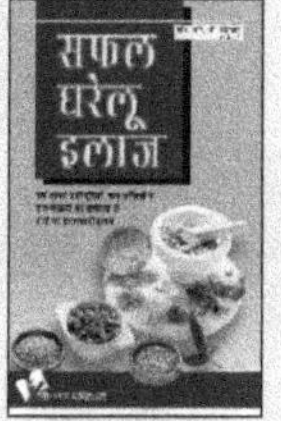
175 pp • ₹ 75

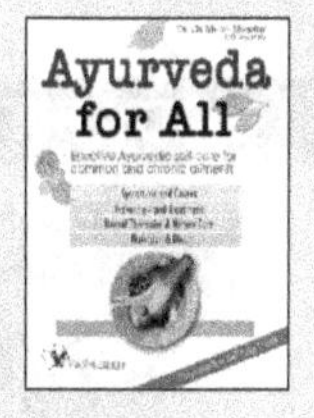
220 pp • ₹ 150

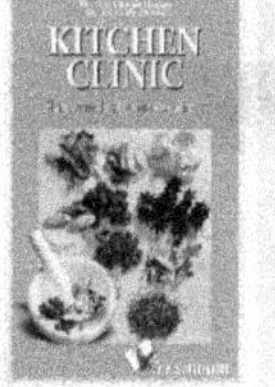
150 pp • ₹ 80

DISEASES & COMMON AILMENTS

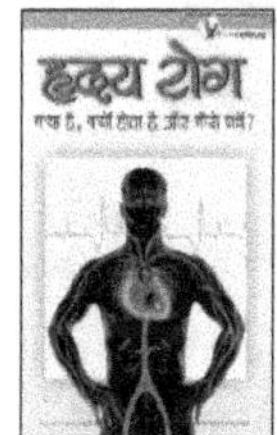
156 pp • ₹ 96

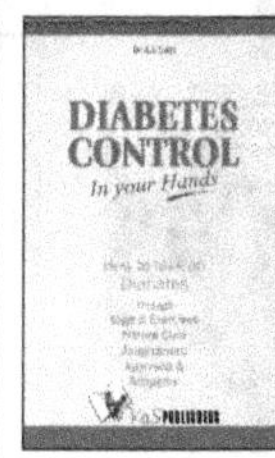
120 pp • ₹ 96

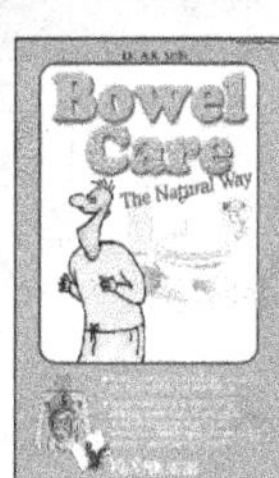
70 pp • ₹ 60

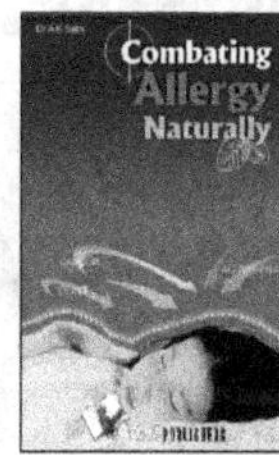
119 pp • ₹ 88

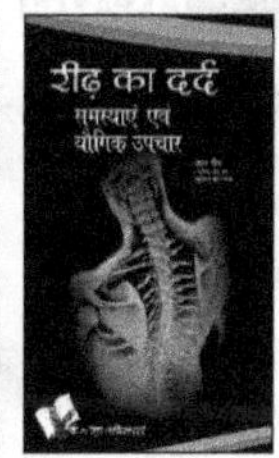
64 pp • ₹ 60

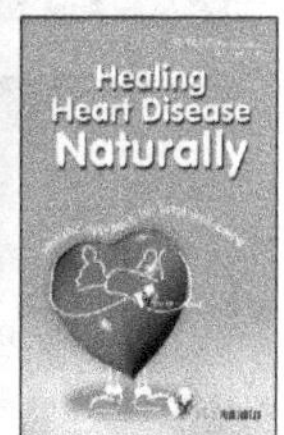
200 pp • ₹ 108

All books available at www.vspublishers.com

YOGA & MEDITATION

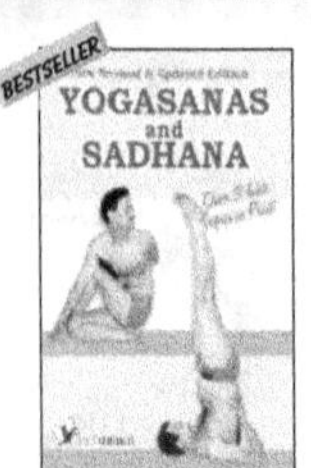

104 pp • ₹ 72

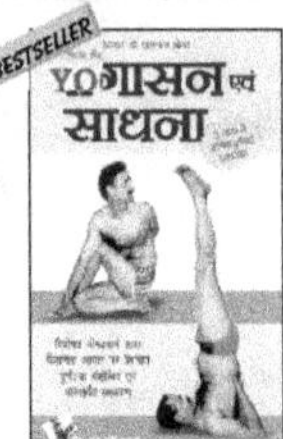

144 pp • ₹ 72

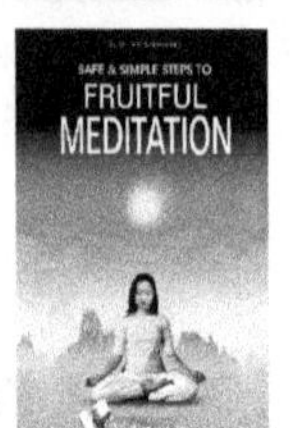

93 pp • ₹ 80

BEAUTY CARE

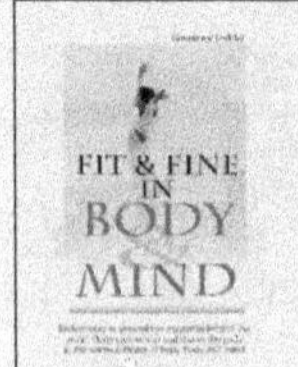

209 pp • ₹ 108

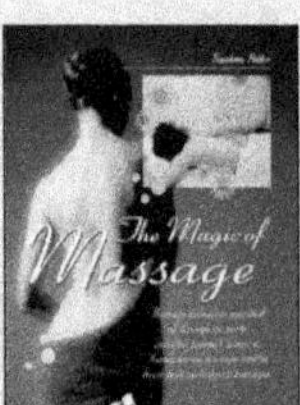

173 pp • ₹ 125

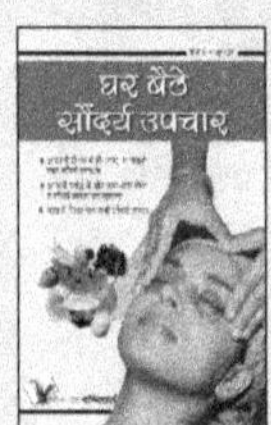

115 pp • ₹ 80

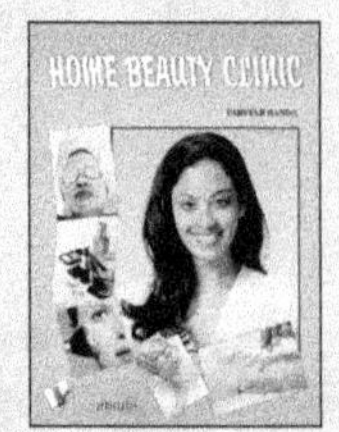

136 pp • ₹ 150

DIET & NUTRITION

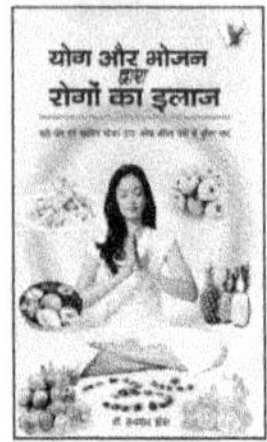

160 pp • ₹ 96

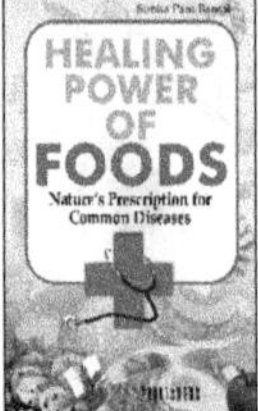

130 pp • ₹ 88

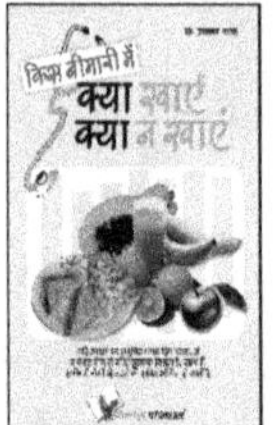

165 pp • ₹ 96

BODY FITNESS

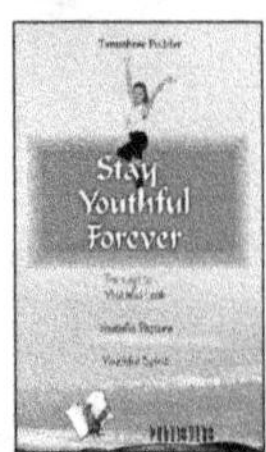

245 pp • ₹ 120

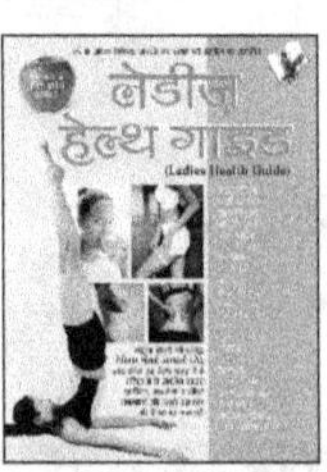

295 pp • ₹ 135

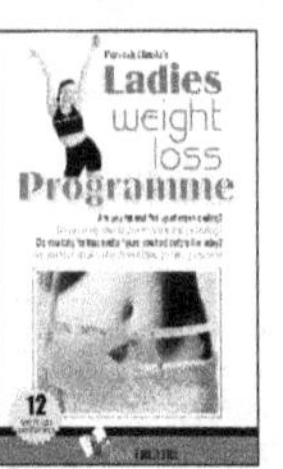

156 pp • ₹ 95

HOUSEKEEPING

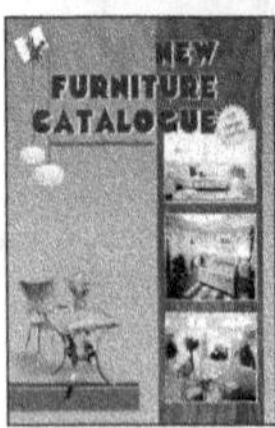

256 pp • ₹ 175

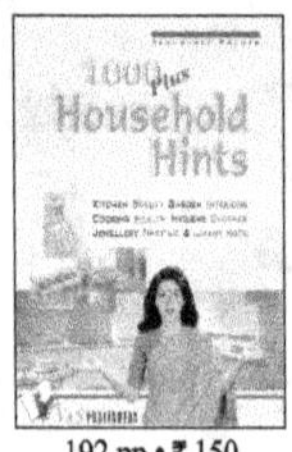

192 pp • ₹ 150

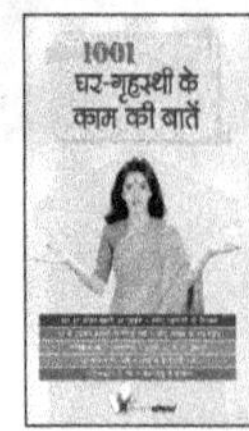

144 pp • ₹ 96

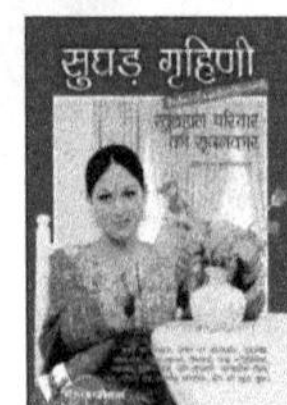

144 pp • ₹ 96

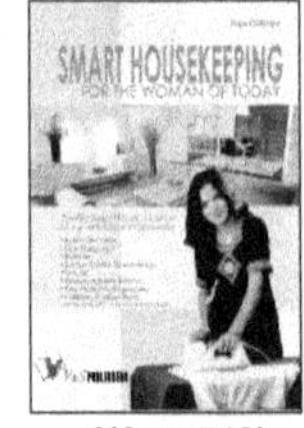

292 pp • ₹ 150

All books available at www.vspublishers.com

SELF IMPROVEMENT

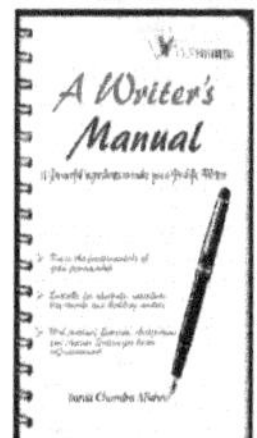

168 pp • ₹ 195

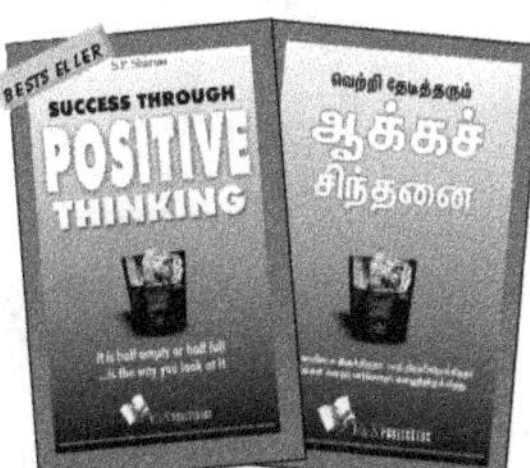

179 pp • ₹ 96

175 pp • ₹ 96
(Tamil)

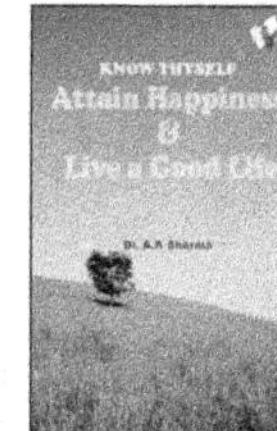

128 pp•₹ 120

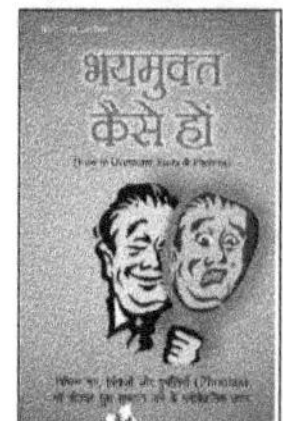

120 pp • ₹ 48

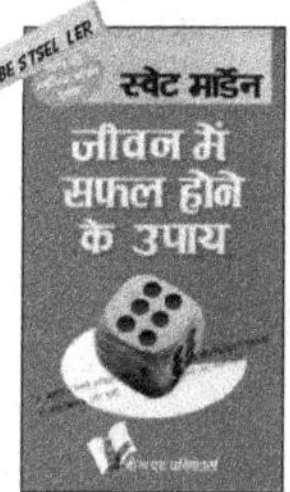

143 pp • ₹ 68

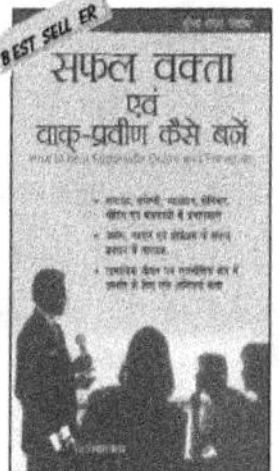

130 pp • ₹ 96

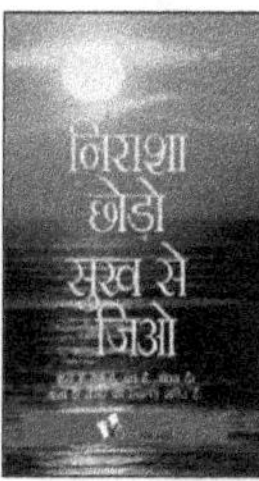

136 pp • ₹ 96

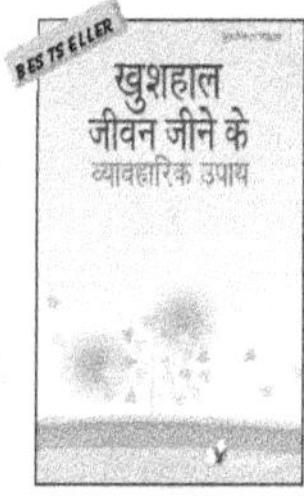

128 pp • ₹ 96

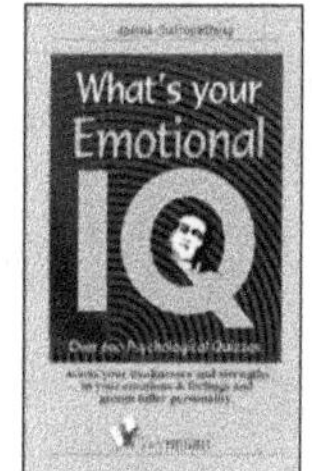

176 pp • ₹ 96

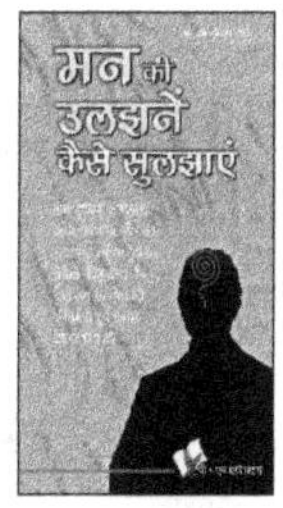

128 pp • ₹ 60

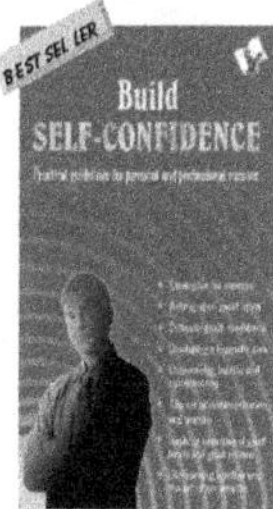

120 pp • ₹ 96

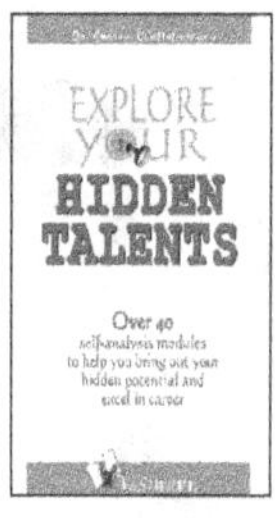

175 pp • ₹ 120

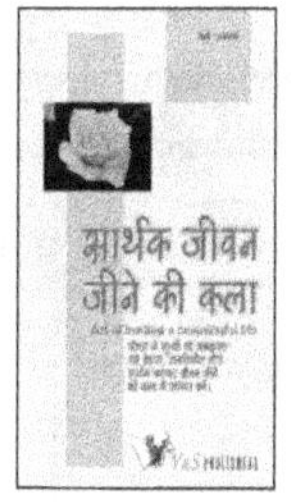

123 pp • ₹ 96

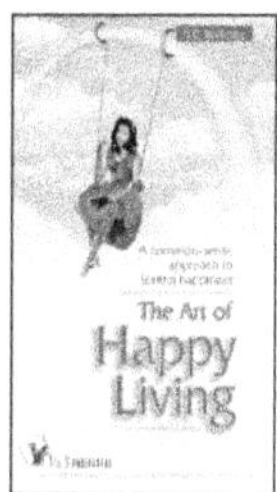

165 pp • ₹ 96

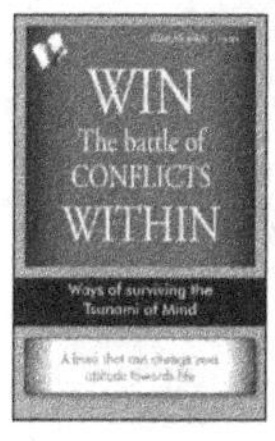

260 pp • ₹ 175

STRESS

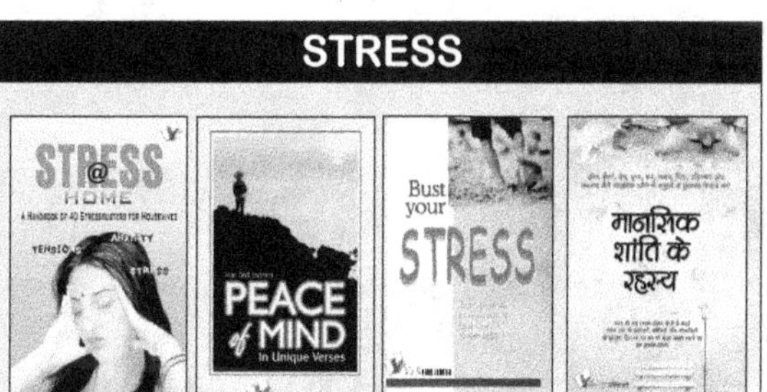

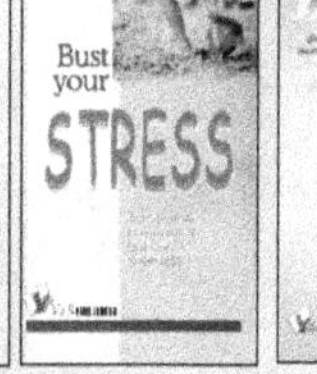

183 pp • ₹ 135

174 pp • ₹ 96

128 pp • ₹ 96

112 pp • ₹ 80

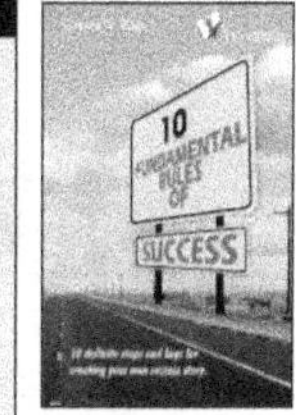

124 pp • ₹ 96

PERSONALITY DEVELOPMENT

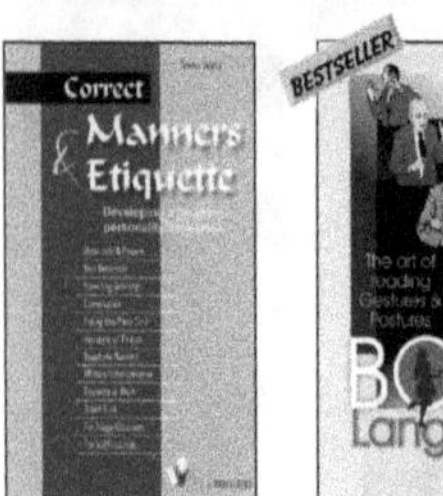

156 pp • ₹ 80

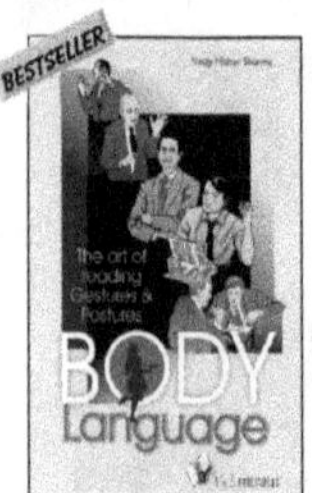

120 pp • ₹ 96

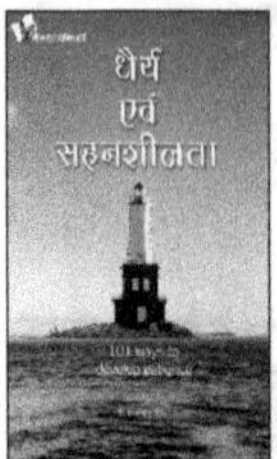

151 pp • ₹ 80

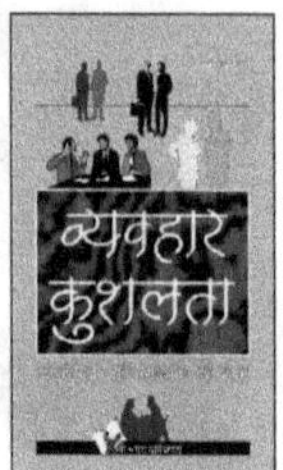

128 pp • ₹ 60

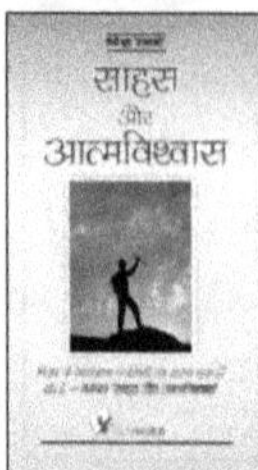

128 pp • ₹ 60

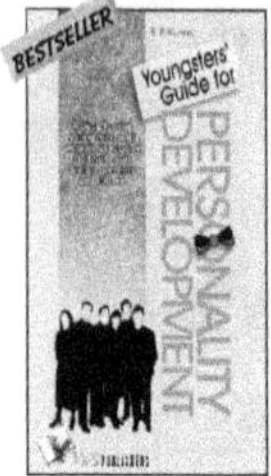

120 pp • ₹ 88

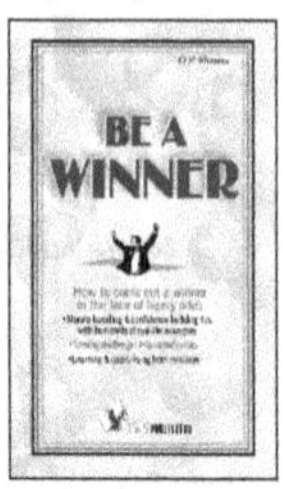

134 pp • ₹ 96

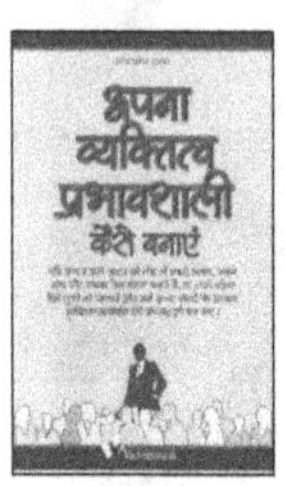

142 pp • ₹ 68

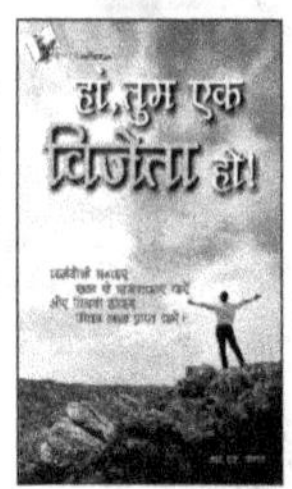

160 pp • ₹ 60

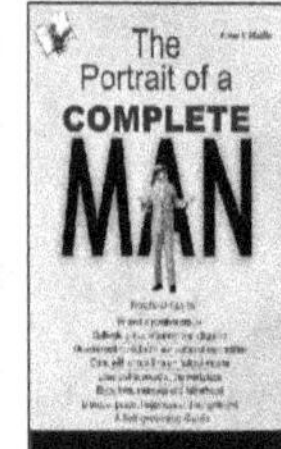

175 pp • ₹ 110

CAREER & BUSINESS

RELIGION

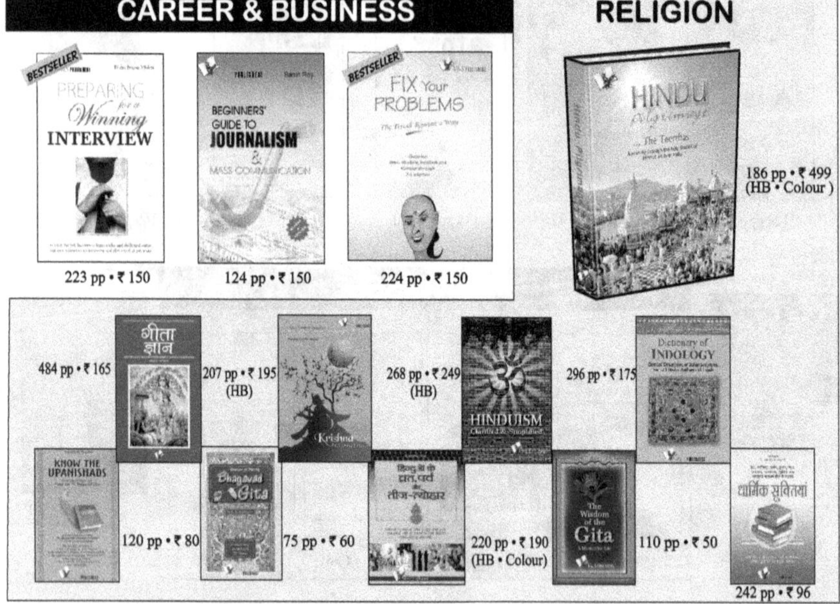

All books available at www.vspublishers.com

STUDENT DEVELOPMENT

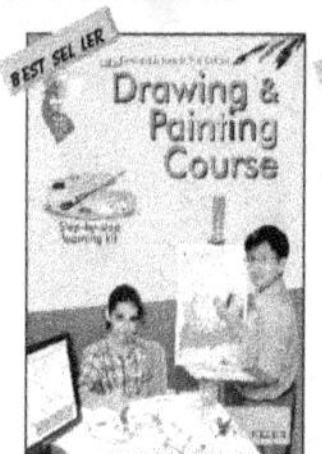

122 pp • ₹ 120
(Free CD)

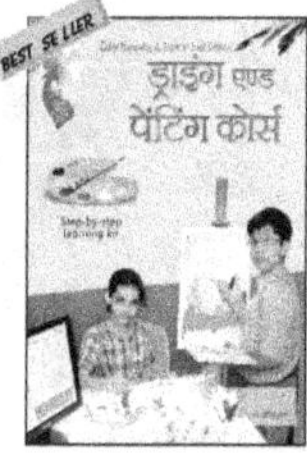

122 pp • ₹ 120
(Free CD)

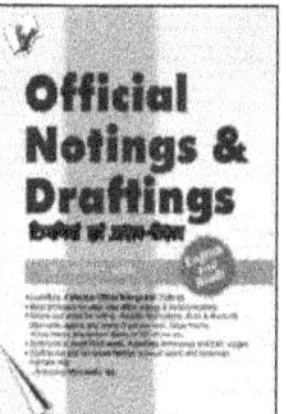

131 pp • ₹ 175

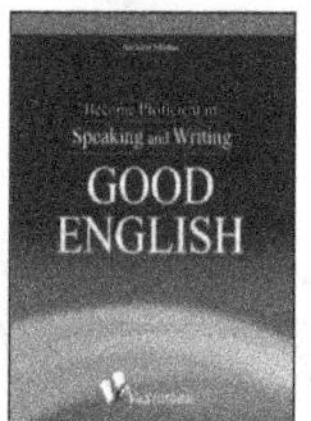

148 pp • ₹ 120

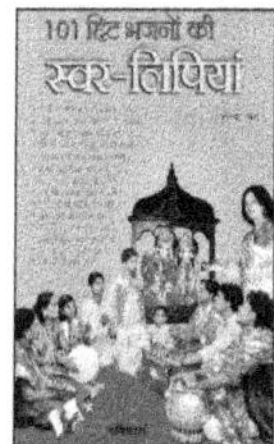

257 pp • ₹ 120

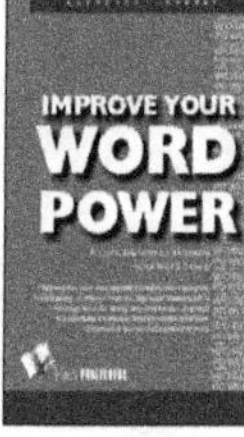

230 pp • ₹ 88

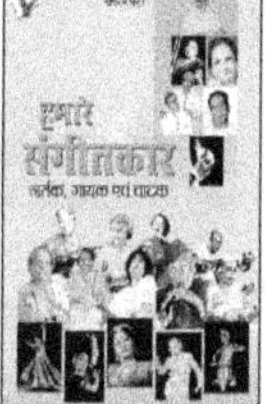

205 pp • ₹ 96

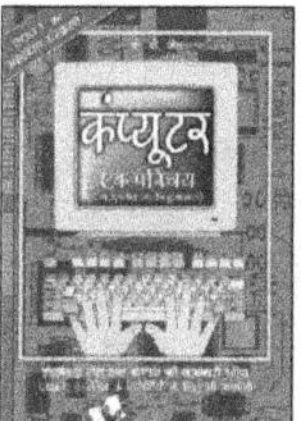

164 pp • ₹ 80

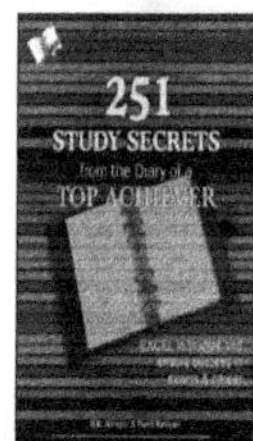

133 pp • ₹ 150

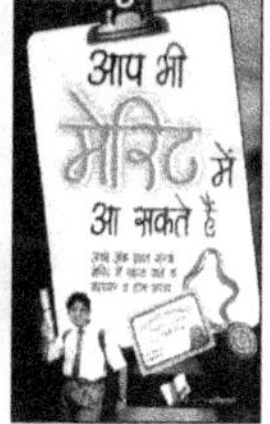

152 pp • ₹ 68

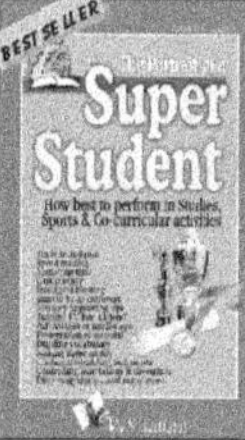

142 pp • ₹ 110

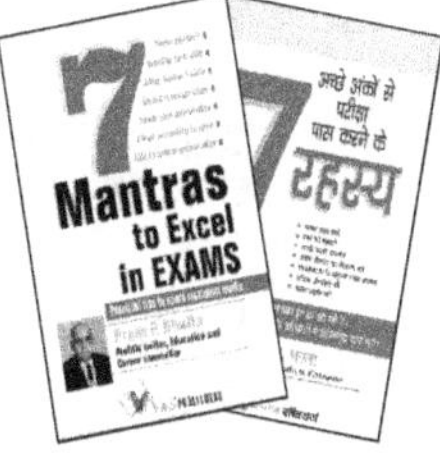

143 pp • ₹ 80 141 pp • ₹ 80

QUOTATIONS

132 pp • ₹ 80

132 pp • ₹ 80

144 pp • ₹ 96

187 pp • ₹ 125

QUIZ / BRAIN TEASERS / PUZZLES

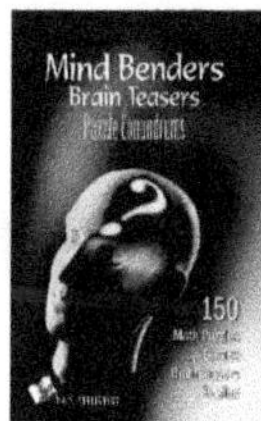

152 pp • ₹110

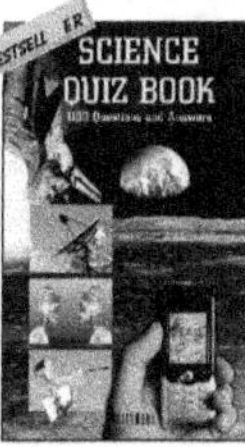

192 pp • ₹ 72

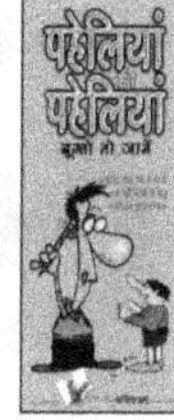

112 pp • ₹ 48

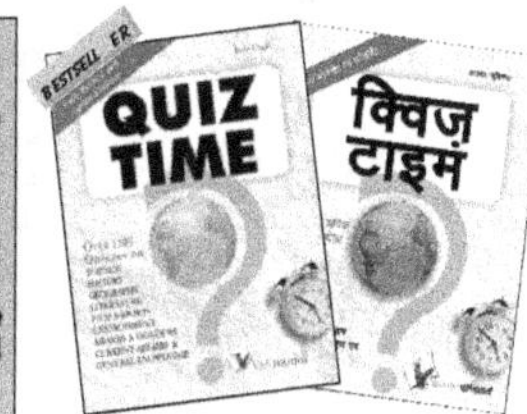

127 pp • ₹ 120 164 pp • ₹ 120

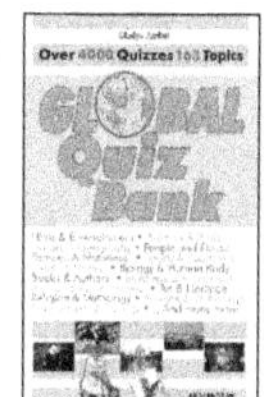

256 pp • ₹ 120

All books available at www.vspublishers.com

FUN / FACTS / MYSTERY / MAGIC

124 pp • ₹ 68 | 104 pp • ₹ 60 | 111 pp • ₹ 72 | 120 pp • ₹ 72 | 120 pp • ₹ 72

112 pp • ₹ 72 | 136 pp • ₹ 100 | 134 pp • ₹ 100 | 136 pp • ₹ 72

CHILDREN STORIES

98 pp • ₹ 96 | 120 pp • ₹ 80

88 pp • ₹ 80 | 128 pp • ₹ 48

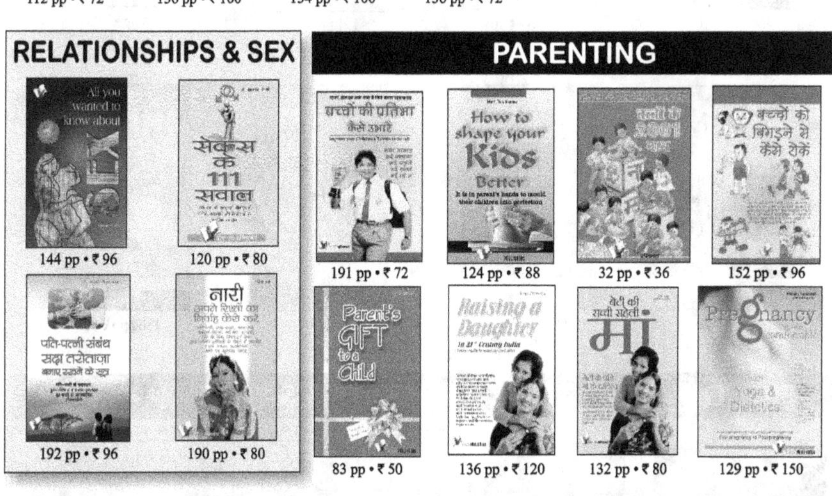

RELATIONSHIPS & SEX

144 pp • ₹ 96 | 120 pp • ₹ 80

192 pp • ₹ 96 | 190 pp • ₹ 80

PARENTING

191 pp • ₹ 72 | 124 pp • ₹ 88 | 32 pp • ₹ 36 | 152 pp • ₹ 96

83 pp • ₹ 50 | 136 pp • ₹ 120 | 132 pp • ₹ 80 | 129 pp • ₹ 150

COOKERY

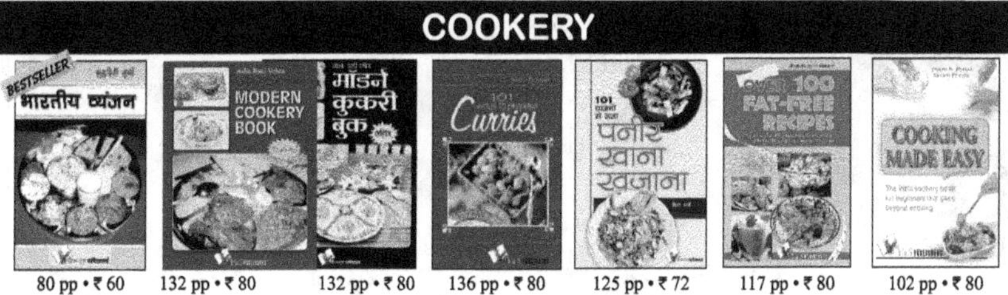

80 pp • ₹ 60 | 132 pp • ₹ 80 | 132 pp • ₹ 80 | 136 pp • ₹ 80 | 125 pp • ₹ 72 | 117 pp • ₹ 80 | 102 pp • ₹ 80

All books available at www.vspublishers.com

ASTROLOGY / PALMISTRY / VAASTU/ HYPNOTISM / OCCULT

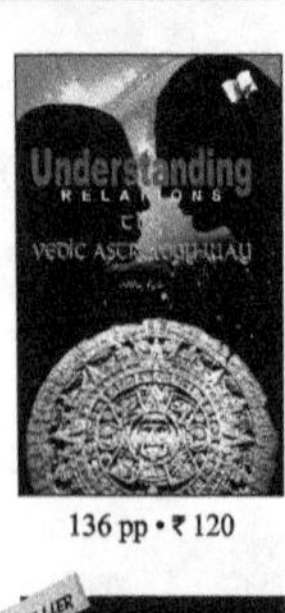

136 pp • ₹ 120

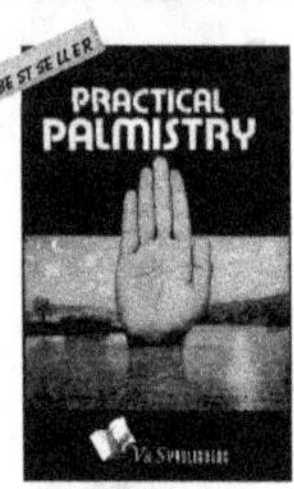

386 pp • ₹ 108

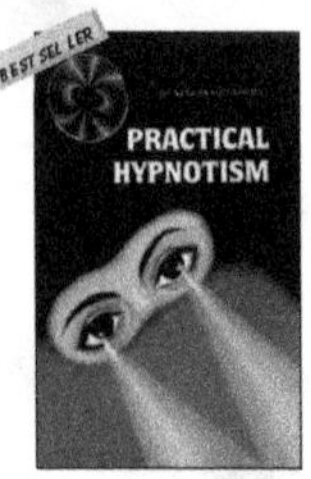

252 pp • ₹ 96

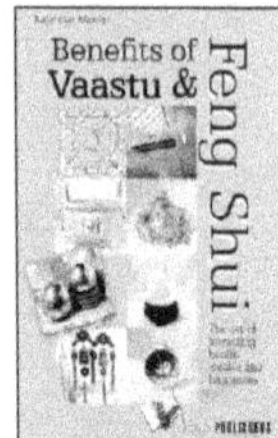

142 pp • ₹ 96

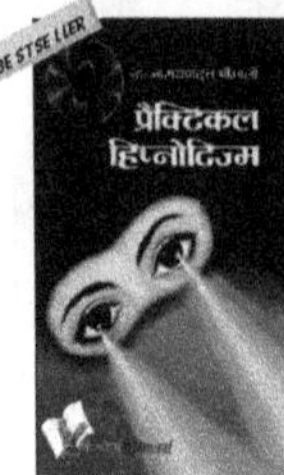

266 pp • ₹ 96

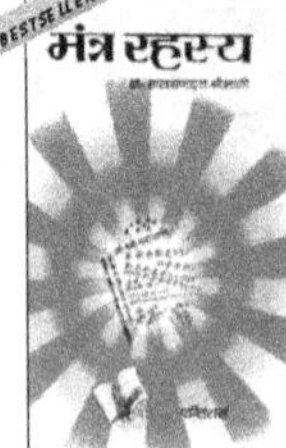

380 pp • ₹ 108

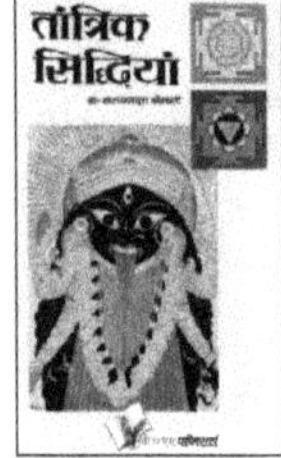

191 pp • ₹ 96

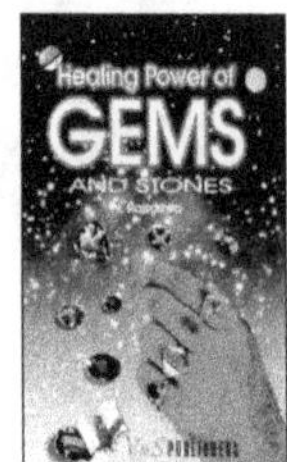

144 pp • ₹ 88

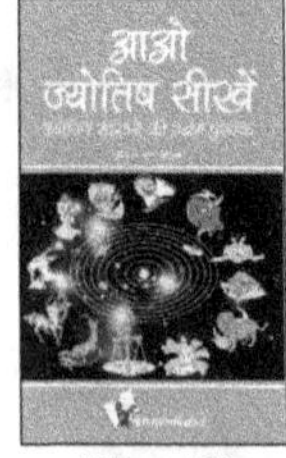

122 pp • ₹ 80

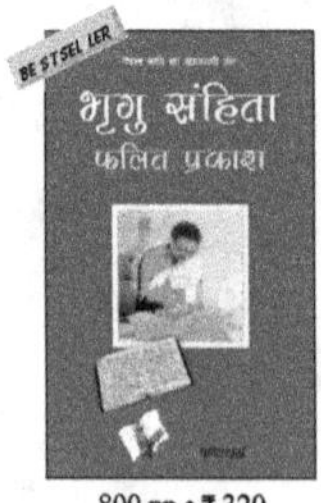

800 pp • ₹ 320
(HB)

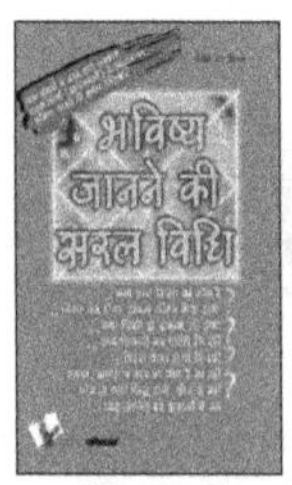

122 pp • ₹ 60

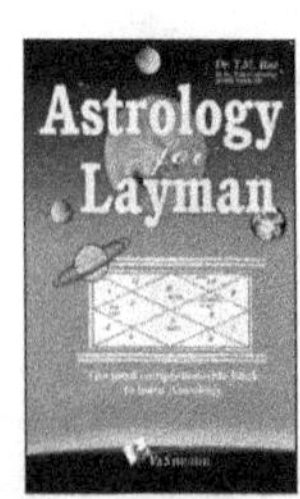

180 pp • ₹ 80

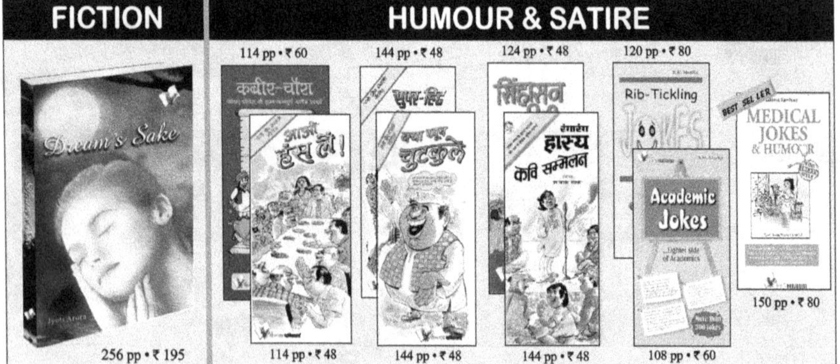

All books available at www.vspublishers.com

www.ingramcontent.com/pod-product-compliance
Lightning Source LLC
Chambersburg PA
CBHW050535270326
41926CB00015B/3237